Natalie Cascella is the CEO and founder of Nuworld Botanicals and author of *Nuworld Botanicals DIY Raw Skincare Recipes*. Natalie has spent the last decade successfully growing her natural skincare brand by selling into major retail stores like Whole Foods Market.

Natalie has a business degree in marketing and has spent the majority of her career working for Fortune 500 companies before leaving her corporate life in 2015 to pursue entrepreneurship full time.

Her flagship retail store is located in downtown Oakville Ontario, Canada and features a unique concept in DIY natural skincare making. Her mission today is to teach natural skincare making and empower people of all ages to take control of the ingredients in their skincare. Natalie can be found teaching DIY skincare classes at her Oakville store and online, and coaching aspiring skincare entrepreneurs at her Masterclass.

Nuworld Botanicals
DIY Raw Skincare Recipes
From Our Store to Your Kitchen!

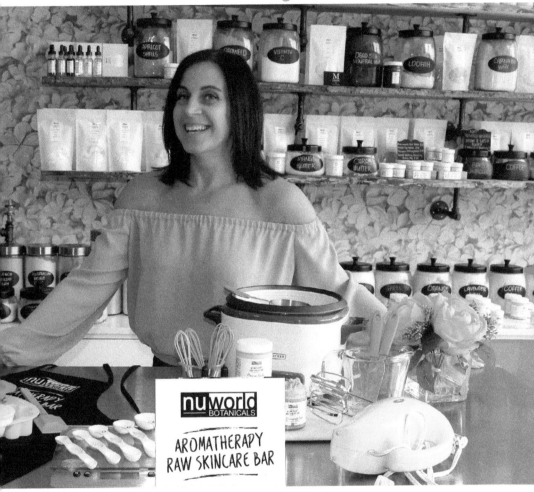

AROMATHERAPY RAW SKINCARE BAR

45 of our Top-Selling Recipes & Ingredients Glossary

Face | Body | Hair | Make-up | Baby

Natalie Cascella
Founder & CEO Nuworld Botanicals

AUSTIN MACAULEY PUBLISHERS™
LONDON • CAMBRIDGE • NEW YORK • SHARJAH

Copyright © Natalie Cascella (2021)

Ordering Information
Quantity sales: Special discounts are available on quantity purchases by corporations, associations, and others. For details, contact the publisher at the address below.

Publisher's Cataloging-in-Publication data
Cascella, Natalie
Nuworld Botanicals DIY Raw Skincare Recipes

ISBN 9781645758532 (Paperback)
ISBN 9781645758525 (Hardback)
ISBN 9781645758549 (ePub e-book)

Library of Congress Control Number: 2021901176
www.austinmacauley.com/us

First Published (2021)
Austin Macauley Publishers LLC
40 Wall Street, 33rd Floor, Suite 3302
New York, NY 10005
USA

mail-usa@austinmacauley.com
+1 (646) 5125767

To all of those hard-working artisan skincare makers making a positive impact on our skin, health, and the environment.

My husband, Johnny, and our children, Nick and Adrianna, for supporting me in pursuit of my dream business ten years ago and in writing this book.

Lana Marconi, R.Ac., my sister and TCM acupuncturist (Marconi Acupuncture), for sharing her knowledge in health and wellness and inspiring my journey.

My parents, Larry and Elisa, for their encouragement and igniting my entrepreneurial spirit.

My incredible team of Master Mixologists, I want to acknowledge your assistance in creating this book, from the recipe trials and tests to the photography and product modelling, you guys rock!

Linda, my graphic designer, there is no way I would have accomplished the feat of completing this book without your skills and expertise.

Julius, for your invaluable contribution and visual media expertise.

My publisher, the entire Austin Macauley team, I am forever grateful for this opportunity you have given me, it means the world.

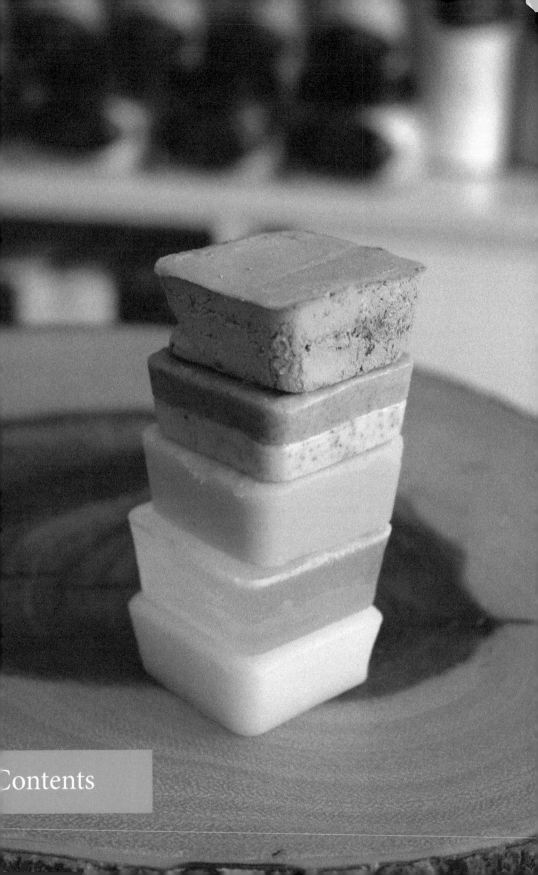

Contents

Hi there, DIY
skincare maker!

My name is Natalie and I'm the founder and CEO of Nuworld Botanicals. For the past ten years, I've been making and selling my own natural skincare products. I've been fortunate to grow my brand by selling into major national retail stores like Whole Foods Market, Chapters Indigo, Well.ca, and Canadian home shopping television channel TSC. I've also created private label skincare for companies in the natural beauty and lifestyle space. In 2016, I decided it was time to open my own retail store—**Nuworld Botanicals Aromatherapy & Raw Skincare Bar.**

I began my DIY natural skincare journey like many of you—from my own kitchen. To this day, I still make all of my skincare products in small batches right inside my downtown Oakville store with the help of my master mixologists. My shop is like a smoothie bar—a treasure trove of raw organic superfood ingredients for custom-blending. I also host DIY workshops and teach a masterclass for aspiring entrepreneurs looking to kick-start their own natural skincare brand.

In this recipe book, I've compiled some of my best-selling skincare recipes that you can whip up in your own kitchen; some recipes are products I've sold in Whole Foods Market! Explore my glossary of organic and vegan skincare ingredients—mix and match ingredients, create, and experiment. You can find most of these ingredients at my Oakville store, and online at nuworldbotanicals.com.

Ready to delve into the world of natural skincare making? Let's begin!

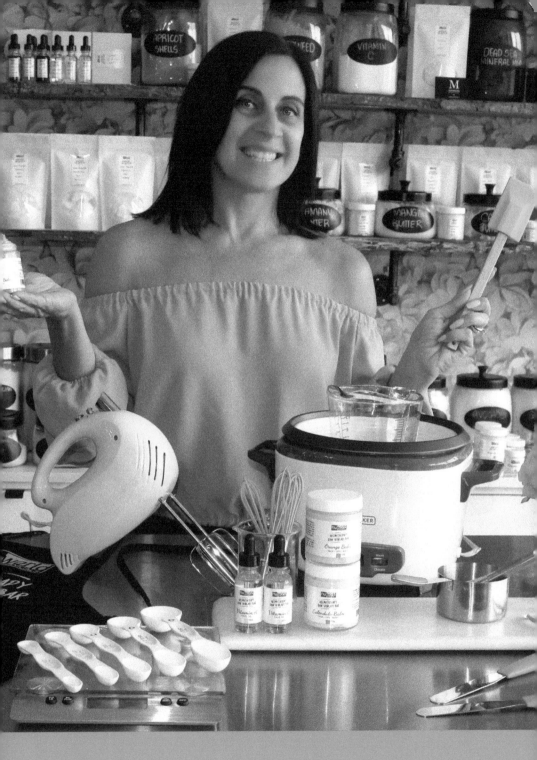

Natalie Founder & CEO

My Journey Into DIY Natural Skincare

I'm a self-taught DIYer. I never had any extended training in aromatherapy nor do I have a chemistry background. What I do have is a passion for healthy living, business training, and an entrepreneurial spirit. I come from a family of entrepreneurs. Growing up, my parents owned and operated several restaurants, homemade Italian with a craft brewery. My father was an amazing chef and even launched his own line of retail pasta sauces and Italian beer. My parents instilled a good work ethic in me, and I believe that helped shape the entrepreneur I am today. After university, I never stayed in the family restaurant business. As much as I enjoyed it, it just wasn't my passion. I would spend the next 20 years working for Fortune 500 companies, in corporate marketing.

My love affair with DIY natural skincare started over a decade ago while doing market research for a wellness fair at my workplace. The research led me to an article by David Suzuki, *The Dirty Dozen Cosmetic Chemicals to Avoid*. That was my aha moment. It got me thinking about my own skin and health concerns—skin rashes, eczema, allergies, and migraines. I had never put two and two together, that maybe what I was putting on my skin could be causing this.

According to Suzuki, the term "fragrance" or "parfum" on a personal care ingredients list usually represents a complex mixture of dozens of harmful chemicals, some 3,000! And many of these unlisted ingredients are irritants that can trigger allergies, migraines, and asthma symptoms. Petrolatum, a mineral oil jelly, is used as a barrier to lock moisture in the skin and is found in a variety of moisturizers, and also in hair care products to make your hair shine. A petroleum product, petrolatum can be contaminated with polycyclic aromatic hydrocarbons (PAHs) and PAHs in petrolatum can also cause skin irritation and allergies.

After that, everything changed. I set out to become a better product label reader. I began to dissect ingredients on my skincare packages. It wasn't easy to navigate, but it was clear to me that brands both conventional and those claiming to be natural, can so easily take advantage of customers aiming for a healthier lifestyle. Despite what a beauty product may claim on its packaging, what lies inside isn't always as "natural" or "clean" as one might hope. I thought there has to be a better way. I decided to delve into natural skincare making.

I picked up some essential oil bottles from my sister Lana, a wellness practitioner (she always had natural remedies around her office) and I bought some basic carrier oils from my local health food store—jojoba and sweet almond. I did some research on skin reparative oils and came across Sea Buckthorn oil. After a few attempts at DIY, I had created my first 100% raw face oil—with less than four ingredients! My sensitive skin never felt or looked better—bye, bye, redness and dry patches. I wanted to tell everyone about it. I set out on a mission to create and replace as many toxic personal care items as I could, and share them with family and friends.

What started out as a personal DIY journey, organically grew into a full-fledged business. In 2009, I started my new company, Nuworld Botanicals. It was a side-hustle for the first few years. The first product line I developed was my Aromatherapy Personals roll-ons. The concept was 12 ready-to-use aromatherapy roll-on remedies, for what ails you. The line was designed for people of all ages who wanted to experience the real benefits of aromatherapy, quickly, easily, and on-the-go. My rollerball vials made it all the way to Whole Food Market stores and jump-started my career as an artisan skincare entrepreneur.

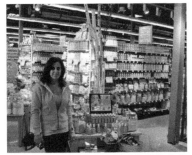

Natalie's products launch into Whole Foods Market Mississauga, Ontario, June 2013

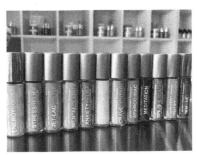

Natalie's signature Aromatherapy Personals Roll-ons

Test Kitchen

TIPS/TECHNIQUES/TOOLS

"The secret to crafting great recipes is practice. Get in the kitchen, grab a few ingredients, and start experimenting. The more you practice, the better it will become."

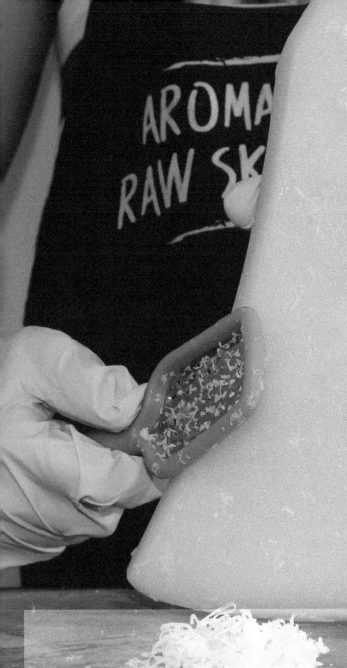

Tip: Say Cheese, Please!

I like to use a basic kitchen cheese grater to shave thin slices off my raw beeswax block. It's just like grating fresh parmesan, and the tiny shreds of wax melt super-fast in the double-boiler.

Tip: Always In-Season

I love working with fruit extract powders like banana, strawberry, and watermelon because they're always in season. They have a reasonable shelf life (about one year) compared to their fresh fruit counterparts which expire in less than a week. They're easier to work with (no blending, mashing, or peeling) and a little goes a long way!

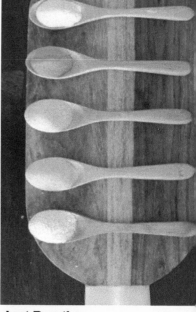

Tip: Just Breathe

Zero-waste solid bars never go out of style, but they will shrink quickly not properly stored. After use, I like keep my bars (shampoo, conditione cleansing, and mask bars) in a drier spot, out in the open where they ca breathe. I find they don't like to be locked up in air-tight containers and they don't like to be left in pooled w for too long either.

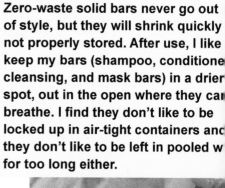

Tip: Glow Oil

You may notice that I use Sea Buckthorn oil...a lot. I love it for its rich Vitamin C content and excellent skin repair qualities. But did you know this bright red berry packs a beta-carotene punch? I'll amp up my face and body oils with a few extra drops of this prized-ingredient for a naturally sun-kissed glow, all year long. I consider Sea Buckthorn oil nature's alternative to a chemical-filled self-tanner.

14

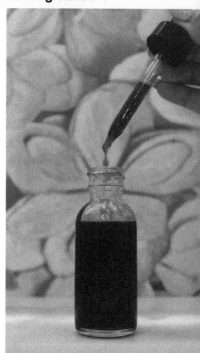

Tip: Travel Light

When I travel, I like to bring my solid bars instead of glass pots (like my lotion bar, mask bar, and hair bars). Bars are zero-waste, ultra-light, and can be easily stored. Ideal for people with on-the-go lifestyles.

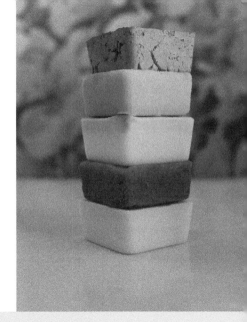

Tip: Eco-Friendly Colors

Raw ingredients like powdered root vegetable extracts (think beetroot and turmeric) and essential oils like blue tansy are not only superstar antioxidants but they do double-duty as natural colorants. No need to use synthetic toxic dyes when mother nature has everything you need.

Tip: Keep It Cool

I store some of my butters, bars, cleansing oils, and facial massage tools in the fridge—not the kitchen fridge but a portable mini skincare fridge. I love the amped up cooling, calming, and soothing effects I get from my chilled products and it looks super-cute on my bathroom counter. Cool, right?

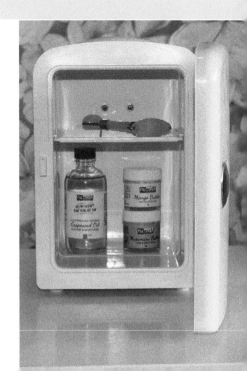

Technique: Quality Check

To check your finished formulations for contamination, there are easy-to-use DIY personal care microbial test kits on the market. Just remember: where there is water, there must a preservative to prevent bacteria, yeast, and mold from growing.
Wearing gloves while working is very important too.

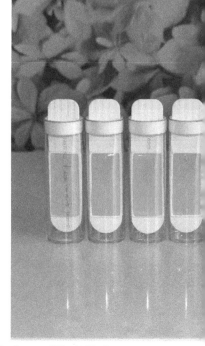

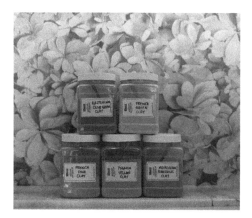

Technique: Mix It Up!

My recipes are meant to be tailored a customized. For instance, you can sw a green "drawing" clay for a milder p clay, or a vitamin E rich oil for a vitan rich oil, depending on your needs. C out my glossary of ingredients and g familiar with the properties. Then, mi and match ingredients to meet your s concerns and scent preference.

Technique: Making Layers

My technique for layering melt and pour soap is fairly straightforward. Make sure the bottom layer has had a chance to cool down, before pouring the second layer. I'll give it about one minute before I pour the next layer. I don't bother with thermometers, nor do I use rubbing alcohol to spray for air bubbles. Check out my scalp detox bars, the lines are not perfectly straight but that's why I love them—they're perfectly imperfect.

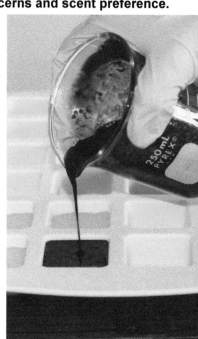

16

Tool: Chop To It!

Trying to melt down one solid bar of melt and pour soap can take forever! I always like to chop up my melt and pour bars into small pieces, before popping them into the double-boiler to melt. I'll use this handy cheese cutter—works like a charm.

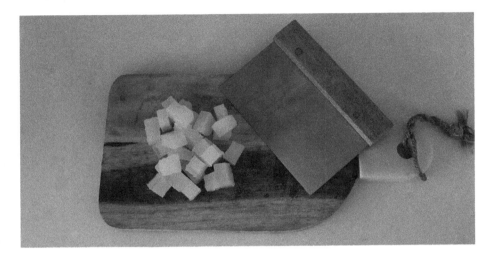

Tool: Double-Boiler Effect

Deciding on a double boiler relies heavily on the way that you'll be using it. For me, it had to be portable, cost-effective, and efficient. I came up with this do-it-yourself double boiler: it's a rice cooker! I simply sit my stainless pots on top to create a double boiler effect. Pop on the lid to help speed up the melting and you're good to go. Works great, travels well. Comes in all sizes too.

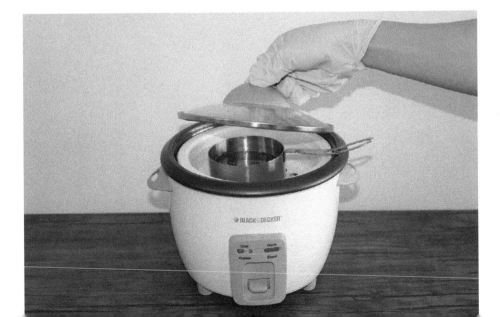

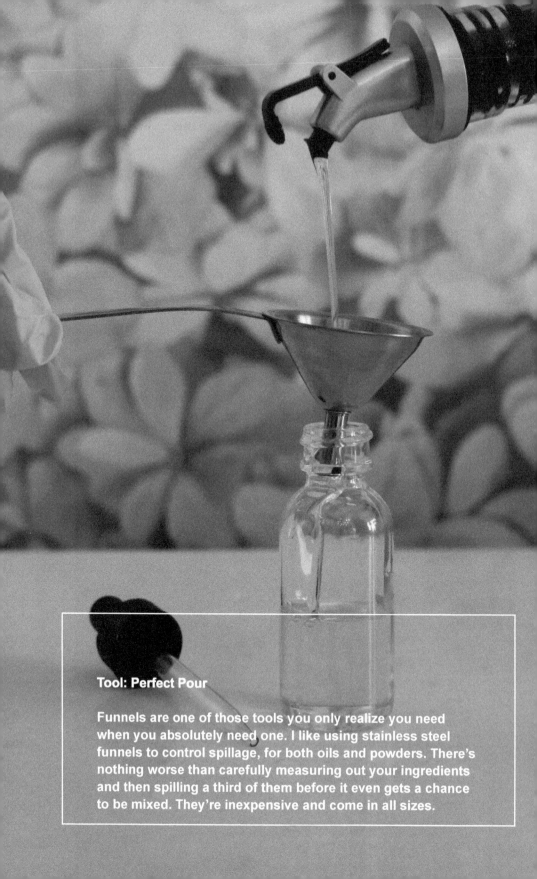

Tool: Perfect Pour

Funnels are one of those tools you only realize you need when you absolutely need one. I like using stainless steel funnels to control spillage, for both oils and powders. There's nothing worse than carefully measuring out your ingredients and then spilling a third of them before it even gets a chance to be mixed. They're inexpensive and come in all sizes.

Tool: Drizzle Me

The secret to that artsy drizzle icing on our artisan cleansing bars is all in the squeeze bottle. The small opening at the tip produces a thin stream of "icing" from start to finish. A basic and inexpensive must-have tool.

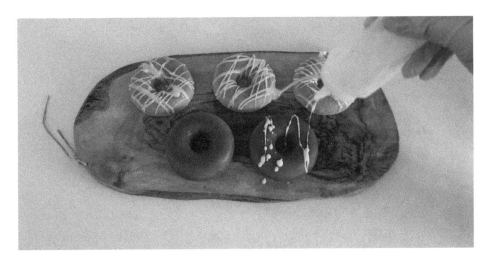

Tool: Pop it!

I love working with silicone molds. They're flexible and bendable, which makes it easier to release solid bars like my shampoo bars. They come in all shapes and sizes—some molds we use serve up 24 bars at once. Silicone molds are also reusable and washable and don't require lining, although I will lay down parchment paper to help pop-out some denser bars, like my clay mask bars.

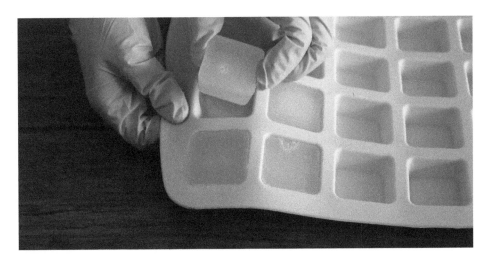

Glossary of Raw Ingredients

Mix and match ingredients to craft the perfect recipe. That's the fun of DIY!

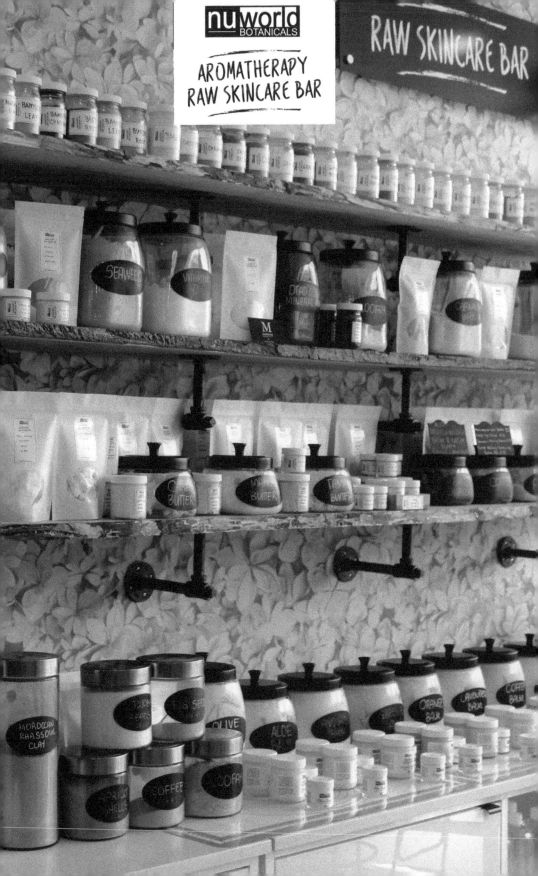

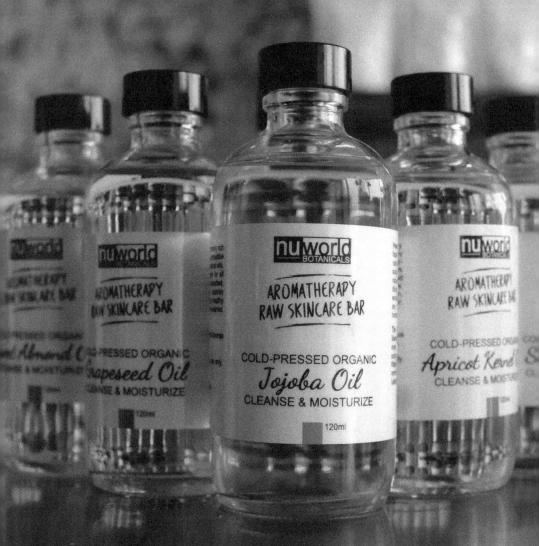

Cold-pressed Carriers

Aloe Vera Oil
Aloe Vera oil contains anti-inflammatory, antibacterial and antioxidant properties. It can help improve acne, promote wound healing and treat sunburns.

Apricot Kernel Oil
Apricot kernel oil is extremely light, yet emollient. High in vitamins A, B and K. Apricot oil helps soothe and heal irritated skin, rejuvenate skin cells and soften fine lines. Vitamin K in this oil can help with dark circles under the eyes.

Argan Oil
Argan oil is one of those oils that falls in the middle of the spectrum—it's not too heavy, not too light—making it perfect to use on all skin types. It's packed with omega fatty acids and vitamin E, all of which work to lightly moisturize your skin and soften dry patches.

Broccoli Seed Oil
Broccoli seed oil is loaded with moisturizing essential fatty acids, vitamin A and linoleic acid. It is nature's alternative to synthetic silicone and is a wonderful ingredient to use in natural haircare products.

Blueberry Seed Oil
Blueberry oil is rich in essential fatty acids, such as omega-3 fatty acid, vitamins A, B complex, C and E. It can help heal skin conditions like eczema,dandruff and psoriasis.

Borage Oil
Borage oil is prized for its high gamma linoleic acid (GLA) content. It's thought that this fatty acid can help reduce inflammation tied to eczema, psoriasis and even arthritis.

Calendula Oil
Calendula oil is a natural oil extracted from marigold flowers and can help soothe sore, inflamed and itchy skin conditions such as eczema, acneand rashes. It's known for its anti-fungal, antioxidant, anti-inflammatory and antibacterial properties.

Camellia Seed Oil

Japanese Camellia seed oil contains high levels of omega-9, proteins, and vitamins. Known as the beauty secret of the Geishas, it helps keep hair healthy, smooth, glossy, and strong. It can also help promote a smoother, firmer skin appearance.

Extra Virgin Organic Coconut Oil

Extra virgin organic coconut oil is an excellent skin moisturizer and softener. Rich in fatty acids, antioxidants, antibacterial, and anti-aging benefits.

Fractionated Coconut Oil

Fractionated Coconut oil is naturally unscented and rich in vitamin E. Works as an all-purpose moisturizer and skin softener. Works well to recondition dry and damaged hair.

Grape Seed Oil

Rich in fatty acids and emollient properties. Soothes away dryness and irritation. Suitable for all skin types, especially acne-prone or oily skin. Grape seed oil is an extremely light carrier oil; it won't clog pores or cause breakouts.

Hemp Seed Oil

Hemp seed oil contains omega-6 fatty acids, a powerful anti-inflammatory that can help calm irritation on the skin, including acne and some conditions like psoriasis, while keeping the skin moisturized.

Jojoba Oil

Jojoba oil is extremely rich in vitamin E and compatible with the skin's own natural oils. A suitable choice for both dry and oily skin types. Beautifully absorbed, it delivers a soft, superbly moisturized finish and healthy complexion.

Marula Oil

Extracted from the nuts of the Marula tree, this is a rare oil that has powerful properties, including protective antioxidants—in fact, while it is similar to the much more famous Moroccan Argan oil, it actually contains 60 percent more antioxidants!

Meadowfoam Seed Oil
Meadowfoam's claim to fame is all about its stability. It is one of the most stable carrier oils available and can help extend the shelf life of other oils. Meadowfoam has wonderful moisturizing and rejuvenating properties.

Olive Oil
Olive oil is a natural humectant that helps attract moisture to dry skin. It contains numerous antioxidants like vitamin E and vitamin K, which helps lighten dark circles under the eyes. Excellent for dry scalp issues too.

Pomegranate Oil
A super-concentrated oil rich in omega-5 (punicic acid). Pomegranate has strong anti-inflammatory and anti-aging properties which help to fend off free radicals.

Raspberry Seed Oil
Raspberry seed oil is rich in antioxidants, like vitamin E and polyphenols. Studies have shown that when applied to the skin, polyphenols protect the skin from ultraviolet radiation and enhance skin cell regeneration, improving skin tone and elasticity.

Rosehip Seed Oil
Rosehip oil is rich in vitamin C, vitamin A, and lycopene. Helps repair the skin's surface and restore elasticity. A good oil to experiment with for under-eye puffiness, dark circles, and scars.

Safflower Oil
Safflower oil is a very light moisturizing oil, readily absorbed by the skin. Softens dry skin, but is especially beneficial for oily skin with its high linoleic acid content. Helps to maintain skin elasticity.

Sweet Almond Oil
Almond oil is renowned for its rich concentration of oleic and linoleic essential fatty acids, making it a popular choice for facial oils and massage oils. Rich in vitamin D, it makes an excellent moisturizer for itchy and inflamed skin.

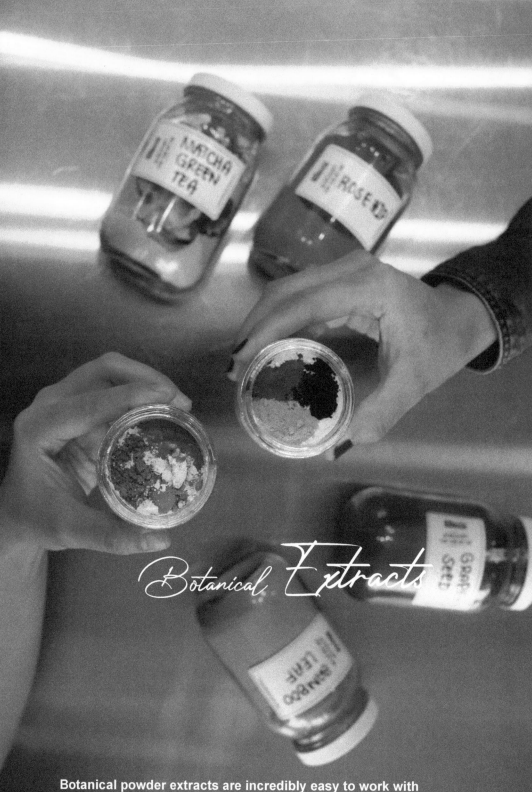

Botanical Extracts

Botanical powder extracts are incredibly easy to work with
and many are probably already in your cupboard.
The DIY possibilities are only limited by your imagination!

Aloe Vera Powder Extract
Aloe vera powder extract is made by organically drying the leaf and inner gel of the Aloe Barbadensis plant. The Aloe leaf is rich in anti-inflammatory properties and can help to alleviate skin ailments like psoriasis, itchy rashes, sunburn, and dryness. The polysaccharides found in Aloe vera powder can even encourage regeneration of skin tissue.

Banana Powder Extract
Banana powder extract contains vitamin A and potassium. It is suitable for dry and sensitive skin.

Cocoa Powder Extract
Cocoa powder extract contains antioxidant properties and flavonoids which help repair and heal sun-damaged skin. Smells just like chocolate!

Cucumber Powder Extract
Cucumber powder extract contains vitamins and minerals essential for healthy-looking skin. It promotes strong cell growth and repair. It also treats swollen or puffy eyes, dark circles, and sunburns.

Honey Powder Extract
Honey powder extract is a natural humectant, which means it attracts and retains water. Rich in antibacterial and anti-inflammatory properties. Helps clean pores, controls surface oils, and calms the skin.

Licorice Root Powder Extract
Licorice root powder extract contains anti-inflammatory properties. It assists with acne, sun-damaged skin, and eczema. It also reduces dark spots, redness, scarring, and blemishes.

Mango Powder Extract
Mango powder extract contains beta-carotene and vitamin C. It's packed with fruit enzymes and alpha hydroxy acids (AHAs), helpful for hyperpigmentation, acne, wrinkles, and dryness.

Matcha Green Tea Powder Extract
Matcha green tea powder extract contains the compound EGCG which gives the powder great antibacterial properties. Aside from its benefits on acne and blemishes, this antioxidant promotes smoother and more supple skin due to its ability to rejuvenate skin cells and support skin structure.

Pineapple Powder Extract
Pineapple powder contains bromelain, a natural enzyme known to exfoliate the skin, unclog pores, and help decrease inflammation. It is also a rich source of natural vitamin C, which makes it an amazing source for brightening and evening skin tone.

Pomegranate Powder Extract
Pomegranate powder extract contains vitamin C and antioxidants that help reduce signs of aging. Helps fight inflammation, treat acne breakouts, and lighten dark spots. It also promotes skin repair and cellular regeneration.

Pumpkin Powder Extract
Pumpkin powder extract has enzymes and antioxidants that offer results similar to gentle alpha hydroxy action. It removes dead, dull cells while nourishing your skin with beta-carotene, leaving it smooth and glowing.

Rosehip Powder Extract
Rosehip powder extract contains beta-carotene (a form of vitamin A) and vitamins C and E. It helps to improve skin elasticity and skin firmness. It can also help reduce the appearance of dark spots.

Sea Buckthorn Powder Extract
Sea Buckthorn powder extract is extremely rich in antioxidant flavonoids and omega fats—in particular omega-7. It is an amazing skin healer and an excellent remedy for sunburn and other types of skin damage. It can protect against free radical damage and encourage collagen production.

Strawberry Powder Extract
Strawberry powder extract is rich in vitamins A and C. It contains salicylic acid that gently exfoliates and removes impurities to brighten skin and shrink pores.

Turmeric Powder Extract
Turmeric powder extract contains curcumin, a potent antioxidant. It helps reduce oil formation and clogged pores. Turmeric also helps fade scars, lighten the skin, and heal wounds.

Wasabi Powder Extract
Wasabi powder extract contains natural antibacterial properties and is rich in potassium, calcium, and vitamin C. It stimulates circulation to the skin and promotes blood circulation.

Watermelon Powder Extract
Watermelon powder extract is known for being rich in vitamin C, amino acids, and lycopene, a powerful antioxidant that's great for sun-damaged skin.It helps UV-stressed skin to rebuild and protect itself from daily toxins.

White Willow Bark Powder Extract
White willow bark is a natural antibacterial and contains astringent properties. Useful for acne, redness, dark spots, and controlling oil sebum production.

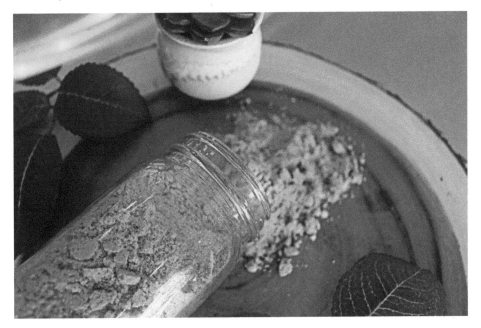

Melt & Pour

With melt and pour soap you can create all types of solid bars- for face, body and hair. It's safe, quick and easy to work with. Plus, you don't need any specialized equipment.

Aloe Vera Melt And Pour Soap
Our Aloe vera melt and pour soap base is a vegetable-based, sulfate-free base. Made using natural Aloe vera, this mild soap base gently cleanses and soothes the skin. Aloe vera is suitable for all skin types, especially dry, damaged, broken, sensitive, and irritated skin.

Argan Melt And Pour Soap
Our Argan melt and pour soap base is a vegetable-based, SLS-free, and non-GMO formula. Commonly known as "Liquid Gold," Argan oil provides fantastic skin softness from the high vitamin E and fatty acid content.

Honey Melt And Pour Soap
Our honey melt and pour soap base is made using real honey. This rich soap base contains natural antioxidants from honey ideal for soothing the skin. Vegetable-based and sulfate-free.

Shea Melt And Pour Soap
Our shea melt and pour soap base is vegetable derived, made using natural ingredients and free from synthetic surfactants and SLS. This melt and pour soap base produces opaque soap bars containing shea butter. Well known for its anti-inflammatory and emollient properties.

Find all of these ingredients in our DIY ingredients shop at nuworldbotanicals.com

Raw Exfoliants

WHITE KAOLIN CLAY

JOJOBA BEADS (vit. E)

FIG SEEDS (vit. A)

APRICOT SHELLS (vit. K)

COFFEE (vit. E)

LOOF

Apricot Shells
Apricot shells are a naturally occurring exfoliant extracted from the seeds of apricot kernels. Apricot shells can help to remove dead skin cells, showing smoother and softer skin. Ideal for stronger exfoliation.

Coffee Seeds
Coffee seed powder is ground from rich coffee beans. It contains chlorogenic acid and may help reduce hyperpigmentation and dark circles under the eyes. The caffeine content in coffee may also be the key to cellulite reduction. Excellent for use in body care products like scrubs and anti-aging face products.

Fig Seeds
Fig seed powder is ground from the fig plant. Rich in vitamin A, it can help reduce the appearance of sunspots, redness, and fine lines. Ideal for anti-aging facial care products.

Jojoba Beads
This natural, non-abrasive exfoliant is often used in exfoliating products designed specifically for sensitive skin. Jojoba beads are polished, round, and smooth. They gently buff away dead skin cells. You can even exfoliate your lips with them!

Loofah
Ground loofah is soft, fine, and sponge-like. It gently exfoliates the skin by polishing away dirt, pollutants, excess oil, and dead cells. An ideal ingredient for body care products like cleansing bars.

Pumice Powder
Pumice powder is a naturally occurring exfoliant from volcanic rocks ground into a powder form. This exfoliating ingredient is ideal for stronger exfoliation. An excellent ingredient for foot scrubs and foot soaps.

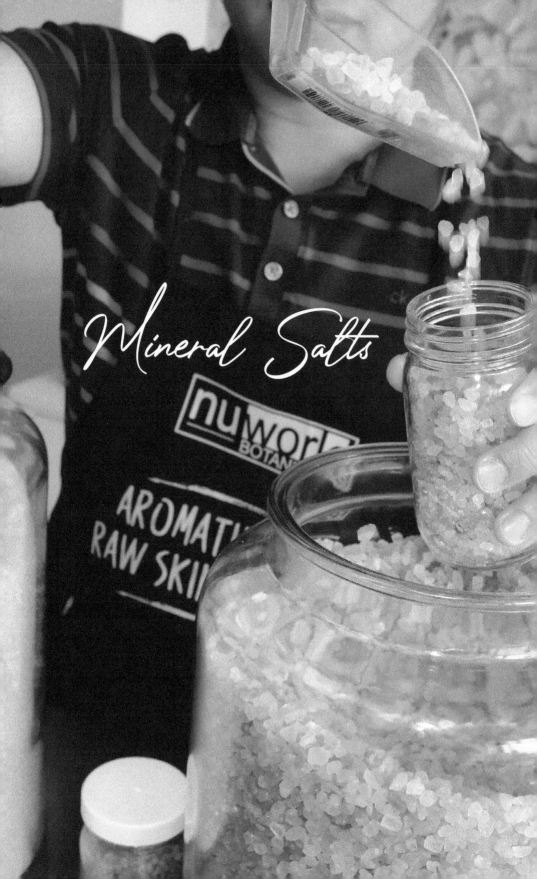

Mineral Salts

Dead Sea Mineral Salt
Dead sea mineral salt contains over 20 health-boosting, skin-loving minerals (which is why we prefer to use salt in our scrubs over sugar). Some examples are: magnesium, which helps speed up healing of the skin; calcium, which enhances skin hydration and can prevent wrinkles; sulfur, which purifies and detoxifies the body; bromide, which relieves muscle cramps and calms the nerves; potassium, which reduces puffiness and water retention; and sodium, which helps to relieve stiff and sore muscles.

Pink Himalayan Salt
Pink Himalayan salt is harvested from the Himalayan mountains. It contains over 84 trace minerals and elements essential to achieving healthier skin. Naturally soothes sore muscles and joints, detoxifies and remineralizes the body back to good health. Used in baths to promote relaxation, reduce stress, and boost energy production. Pink Himalayan salt has the same consistency similar to a coarse salt.

Many of the raw ingredients we use have a shelf life of 1 to 2 years, making them super easy to work with.

FRENCH GREEN CLAY

FRENCH PINK CLAY

AUSTR BEIG CLAY

Mineral Clays

Bentonite Clay
Bentonite clay is able to bind to and extract bacteria and toxins living on the surface of the skin and within the pores. It can help to calm skin irritations, reduce the outbreak of blemishes, and alleviate redness.

Dead Sea Mineral Mud
Dead sea mineral mud draws out impurities and releases beneficial minerals into your skin. Tightens and tones the complexion, balances moisture levels, and promotes elasticity.

French Green Clay
French green clay's unique composition includes iron, silica, magnesium, sodium, and potassium. This clay quickly absorbs and removes impurities from the skin, revealing the fresh surface of the skin to provide a healthy-looking glow. When the clay dries on the skin, it causes pores to tighten and the skin starts to feel firm, toned, and refreshed.

French Pink Clay
French pink clay has a unique composition that includes kaolinite, iron, illite, montmorillonite, and calcite. It gently cleanses the skin and sloughs off dead skin cells to create an overall refreshed appearance.

French Yellow Clay
French yellow clay is made up of fine mineral particles and iron oxides. It is a very mild clay that can be used on dry or sensitive skin.

Kaolin White Clay
Kaolin white clay is a very mild and light clay. It gently exfoliates and cleanses the skin without drawing oils. Perfect for dry and sensitive skin types.

Moroccan Rhassoul Clay
Moroccan rhassoul clay is quarry mined from ancient deposits deep beneath the Atlas Mountains in Morocco. It is sun-dried and untreated. Rhassoul contains a high percentage of silica and magnesium and can help reduce dryness and flakiness of the skin while improving the texture. Rejuvenates and detoxifies.

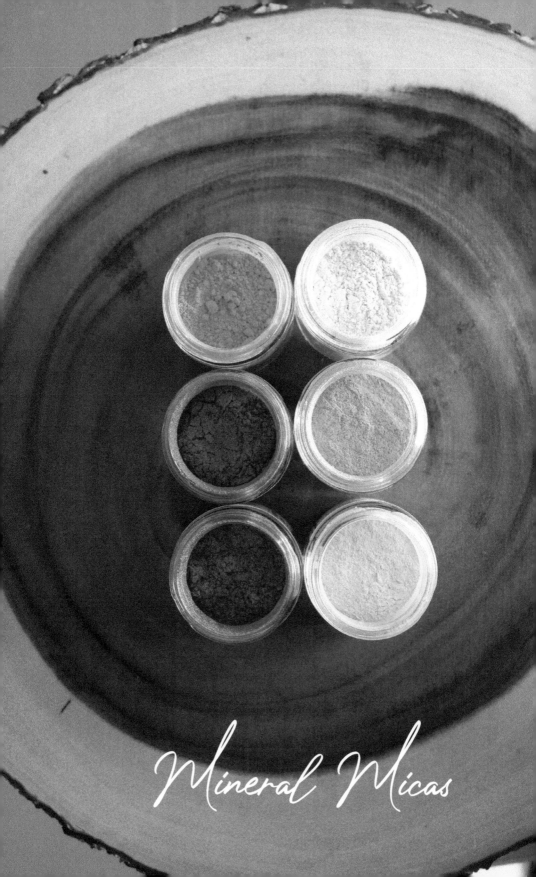

Mineral Micas

Mineral Mica Powder
Mica minerals naturally occur in the earth and are crushed into a
fine powder. Natural mica powder is used to reflect light and create a
pearlescent effect on the skin. Micas come in a range of beautiful shades.
Commonly used in mineral makeup or cosmetics.

Natural Mineral Pigments
Mineral pigments come from various quarries around the world including
France and the Blue Ridge Mountains of Virginia. They contain cosmetic
grade iron oxide. Some have been fired to get their vibrant color.
Available in a range of beautiful shades like burnt umber, ultramarine
blue, yellow, and violet. Commonly used in mineral makeup or cosmetics.

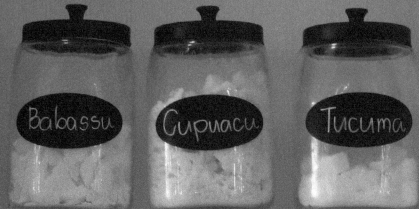

Raw & Exotic Butters

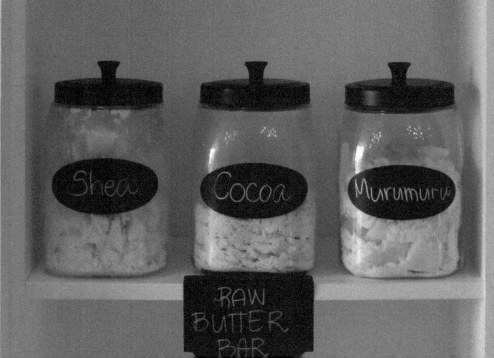

Babassu

Cupuacu

Tucuma

Shea

Cocoa

Murumuru

RAW
BUTTER
BAR

Aloe Butter
Aloe butter is soothing and cooling and rich in vitamins C and E. Perfect for very dry or sensitive skin, sun-damaged skin, and sunburns.

Babassu Butter
Babassu butter is cold-pressed from sustainable kernels of the Amazon-native Babassu Palm. It is high in lauric and myristic acids and vitamin E. A gentle moisturizer for sensitive, dry, and oily skin. It also softens hair and restores hair strength and elasticity.

Carrot Butter
Carrot butter is rich in beta-carotene, vitamins C and E, and essential fatty acids. These nutrients help improve skin tone, texture, and elasticity.

Cupuacu Butter
Cupuacu butter comes from a cupuacu fruit tree native to the northern Amazon. Known as nature's vegetable lanolin, it has a high capacity to retain water and prevent moisture loss. The high amount of vitamin E in cupuacu butter offers a certain amount of protection from the damaging UV rays from the sun.

Mango Butter
Mango butter is cold-pressed from the mango seed grown in tropical climates. Rich in antioxidants and vitamins A and E that restore and maintain moisture in the skin. It also promotes cell regeneration and treats the appearance of wrinkles.

Murumuru Butter
Murumuru butter has lauric, myristic, and oleic acids which are very beneficial for hair. Known as nature's vegetable silicone, this butter can treat dry itchy scalp issues, eliminate frizz, and repair split ends at a very fast rate.

Shea Butter
Shea butter is cold-pressed from the sustainable barks and leaves of karate trees native to Africa. It has high levels of vitamins A and E. It is also renowned for its skin-softening and moisture-retaining ability.

Tamanu Butter
Tamanu butter is cold-pressed from sustainable nut kernels of the Tamanu tree in the South Pacific. Rich in antioxidant, anti-inflammatory, and anti-bacterial properties. It regenerates the skin and heals wounds, burns, and cuts.

Jars on top shelf:

PUMPKIN | PINE-APPLE | ROSEHIP | SEAWEED | STRAW-BERRY | | SPIRULINA |

EMULSIFYING WAX

BEESWAX

Waxes Antioxidants Preservatives

CARNAUBA WAX

CANDELILLA WAX

Beeswax
Beeswax is a natural wax produced by honey bees. It contains vitamin A for cell repair and anti-inflammatory properties which help promote wound healing.

Candelilla Wax
Candelilla wax is a plant-based wax and a suitable vegan alternative to beeswax. It adds shine and smoothness to the finished product and is less sticky than beeswax.

Carnauba Wax
Carnauba wax is a vegetable wax valued for its hardness and high melting temperature. It is used primarily as a thickening agent.

Emulsifying Wax
Used as an ingredient in natural and organic cosmetics to keep oils and liquids from separating. Look for one that is PEG-free, gluten-free, plant-based, and preferably approved by Ecocert.

Natural Preservative (paraben-free)
Any product with water in it will require a full-spectrum preservative. Leucidal® Liquid Complete is our natural preservative of choice—it is effective at preventing the growth of bacteria and fungi, including yeast and mold. While the majority of our skincare products are raw, there are some recipes where a water element is used. If you plan on using up your water-based product within 2–3 days, a preservative won't be required.

Sea Buckthorn Oil (vitamin C)
Sea Buckthorn oil is the single highest plant source of natural vitamin C. Also rich in vitamin E, fatty acids, and essential amino acids, along with beta-carotene which gives it a bright berry color.

Vegetable Glycerin
Vegetable glycerin is a clear, odorless humectant with emollient properties. It can soften the skin and assist the skin surface to retain moisture. Look for one that is GMO-free and plant-based.

Vitamin E (Tocopherol)
Vitamin E (MT-50) is a professional use antioxidant with a full spectrum of tocopherols. It can be used to extend the shelf life of oils and slow the oxidization of essential oils.

Essential Oils

We Love for Skincare

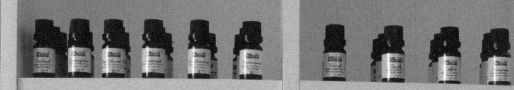

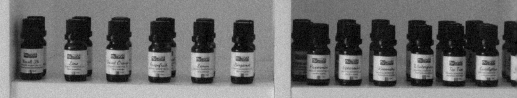

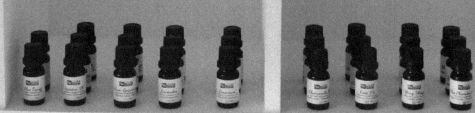

Blue Tansy Essential Oil
Blue tansy essential oil is a powerful anti-inflammatory, suitable for skin conditions like eczema, acne, and rosacea. Due to its chamazulene content, blue tansy essential oil is very dark blue in color.

Frankincense Essential Oil
Frankincense essential oil is a powerful astringent, meaning it helps protect skin cells. It can be used to help reduce acne, scars, stretch marks, blemishes, and the appearance of large pores and wrinkles.

Lavender Essential Oil
Lavender essential oil helps to restore the skin's complexion and can reduce acne due to its antimicrobial properties. It can also help cleanse your skin and lessen redness and irritation. A good choice for all skin types.

Lemon Essential Oil
Lemon essential oil can help lighten dark spots and reduce the appearance of fine lines and wrinkles. It is rich in anti-fungal and astringent properties. Great for combination and oily skin types.

Neroli Essential Oil
Neroli essential oil is a powerful antibacterial, anti-inflammatory, and antiseptic oil that is great for soothing damaged or irritated skin, healing scars, improving circulation, and reducing lines and wrinkles. Also good for fading stretch marks. A good choice for combination, mature, and sensitive skin.

Orange Essential Oil
Orange essential oil contains high levels of vitamin C which help protect and heal the skin. It can also boost circulation, promote collagen production, decrease wrinkles, and fight free radical damage.

Rose Essential Oil
Rose essential oil has been used in beauty treatments for thousands of years. It is effective against acne breakouts and can help reduce redness and dry skin. It is extremely soothing for sun-damaged and sensitive skin.

Essential Oils

We Love for Haircare

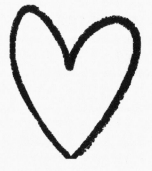

Cedarwood Essential Oil
Cedarwood essential oil is extremely good against seborrheic eczema. It can regulate sebum production and kill the bacteria that cause the infection. Cedarwood deserves a top spot on your list of essential oils for hair.

Chamomile Essential Oil
Chamomile essential oil is a soothing oil that has excellent anti-inflammatory properties. It can relieve an itchy and scaly scalp from dermatitis, psoriasis, or dandruff. Chamomile oil conditions the hair and protects it from the damage inflicted by environmental pollutants.

Clary Sage Essential Oil
Clary sage essential oil regulates oil production and can help control dandruff. It can be used for both dry and oily scalps. You can use it on curly and frizzy hair to make it more manageable.

Lime Essential Oil
Lime essential oil contains antibacterial and antiseptic properties which can help treat and prevent scalp issues like dandruff. It also helps promote healthier hair, providing silky smooth strands.

Peppermint Essential Oil
Peppermint essential oil has a cooling effect we are all familiar with. When applied to the skin, it improves blood flow to the area. This property is very useful for rejuvenating hair follicles and promoting hair growth. Its cleansing action opens up clogged pores and encourages the normal flow of skin oils, making it ideal for people with dry scalp.

Rosemary Essential Oil
Rosemary essential oil is an invigorating oil that can encourage blood circulation in the scalp, stimulating the hair follicles. It has anti-dandruff action and it is best suited for people with oily hair.

Tea Tree Essential Oil
Tea tree essential oil has natural antiseptic, antibacterial and antifungal properties. It works deeply to unclog hair follicles and relieve dryness. Considered the number one natural remedy for dandruff and scalp acne.

Ylang-Ylang Essential Oil
Ylang-Ylang essential oil can help improve hair texture, reduce hair breakage, and stimulate sebum production. Ideal for those with dry scalp issues.

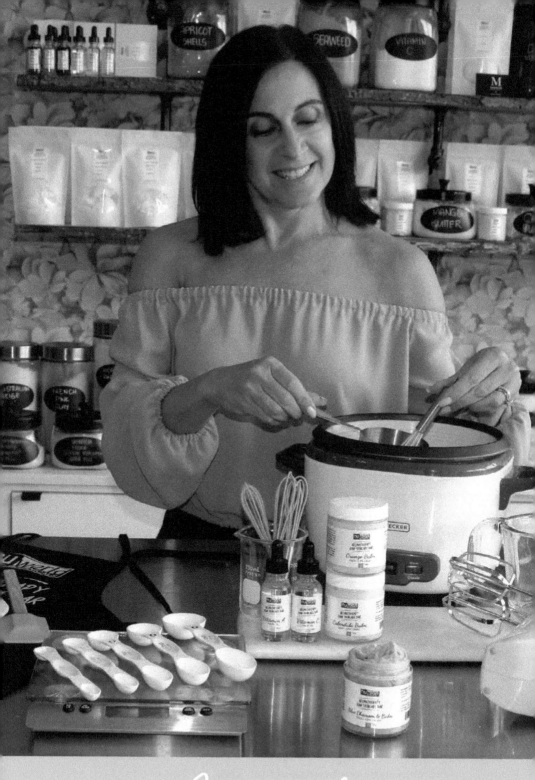

Simple Kitchen Tools

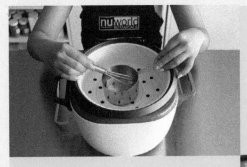

**Double-Boiler
(or a rice cooker!)**

Electric Mixer

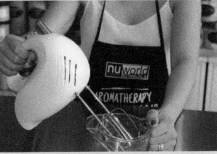

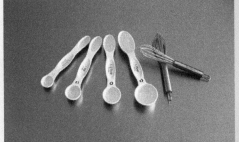

**Measuring spoons
and whisks**

Beakers and a scale

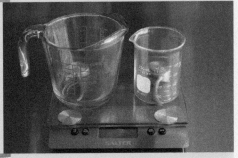

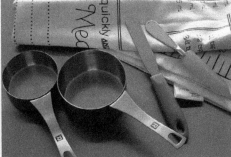

Raw Bodycare Recipes

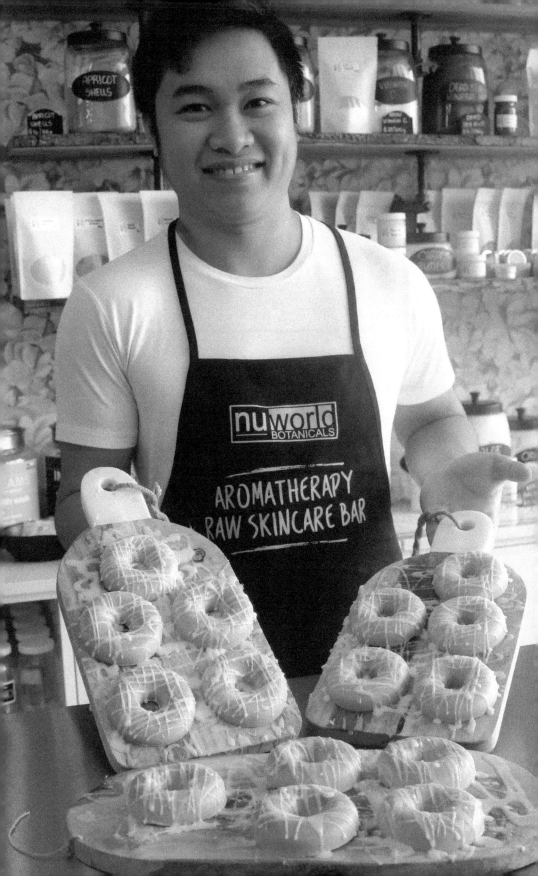

Matcha-Lime Mineral Bath Fizz

Our luxurious bath bomb, but in a jar! Instantly replenishes lost minerals, hydrates the skin, and fizzes just like our traditional bath bomb. Free from toxic SLS, synthetic dyes, coloring, and glitter.

Raw Ingredients:

60 g sodium bicarbonate
30 g citric acid
30 g arrowroot powder
20 g dead sea mineral salt (ultra-fine)
10 g pink Himalayan salt
1/2 tsp kaolin white clay
1/2 tsp matcha green tea powder extract
15 ml safflower oil
8–10 drops lime essential oil

Kitchen Tools:

You will need a bowl, measuring spoon, scale, gloves, and a jar.

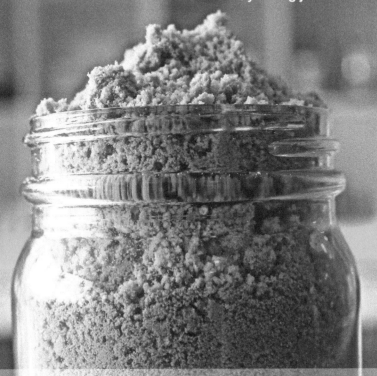

Method:

1. In a large bowl, combine all dry ingredients—sodium bicarbonate, citric acid, arrowroot powder, pink Himalayan salt, dead sea salt ultra-fine, clay, and botanical extract.

2. Wearing gloves, mix well with your hands making sure the mixture is clump-free.

3. Add in the liquid ingredients—safflower oil and essential oils and mix well together.

4. Transfer mixture into the jar

Whipped Rosehip-Strawberry Body Butter

Make our creamy rich body butter from scratch. Brighten your skin (and your day) with this whipped concoction of antioxidant fruit heaven.

Raw Ingredients:

20 g shea butter
10 g cocoa butter
20 ml sunflower oil
5 ml raspberry oil
110 ml distilled water
1/2 tsp rosehip powder extract
1/2 tsp strawberry powder extract
15 g emulsifying wax
5 ml natural preservative (i.e., Leucidal® Liquid Complete)
30 drops essential oil
2 drops sea buckthorn oil
2 drops vitamin E

Kitchen Tools:

You will need a double boiler, metal pots, scale, beakers, measuring spoons, spatula, whisk, an electric mixer, and a jar.

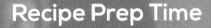

Recipe Prep Time

Prep Time: 15 minutes
Set Time: 20 minutes
Qty: 120 g jar

Method:

1. In a double boiler, gradually melt the shea and cocoa butter. Add in the emulsifying wax.
2. Once melted, add in sunflower oil and raspberry oil.
3. In a separate pot, heat up distilled water. Add in the rosehip and strawberry extract.
4. Once the butters and emulsifying wax are melted, remove from heat and pour in a beaker or Pyrex.
5. Remove the distilled water containing extracts from heat and pour into a separate beaker.
6. Gradually add the distilled water with extracts to the oil phase and continue to whisk.
7. Let cool for about five minutes.
8. Add in vitamin E, natural preservative, essential oils, and whisk.
9. Add sea buckthorn oil. Whisk.
10. Pop in the fridge for about 20 minutes to thicken.
11. Fluff it up with an electric hand mixer.
12. Transfer mixture into the jar.

Vegan Cupuacu-Orange Lotion Bar

This zero-waste, package-free solid body lotion bar is ultra-hydrating with a hint of sun-protection from raspberry seed oil. Glides on and sinks into the skin.

Raw Ingredients:

10 g shea butter
10 g cupuacu butter
1 tbsp extra virgin organic coconut oil
7 g vegan candelilla wax
1 tsp raspberry oil
1 drop sea buckthorn oil
20 drops orange essential oil
1 drop vitamin E

Kitchen Tools:

You will need a double boiler, metal pots, scale, beaker, measuring spoons, spatula, a whisk, and silicone molds.

Recipe Prep Time

Prep Time: 15 minutes
Set Time: 20 minutes
Qty: 2 x 30 g bar

Method:

1. In a double boiler, gradually melt the butters, extra virgin coconut oil, and candelilla wax.
2. Once melted, add in the raspberry oil. Whisk.
3. Transfer into beaker or Pyrex; add in the sea buckthorn oil, essential oil, and vitamin E.
4. Whisk and work quickly as the mixture solidifies quickly.
5. Pour into silicone molds.
6. Pop in the fridge for about 20 minutes to set faster.
7. Allow bar to solidify thoroughly before using.

Vanilla-Cocoa Mineral Bath Bomb

A bath bomb that replenishes lost minerals, hydrates the skin, and smells good…naturally! Free from toxic SLS, synthetic dyes, coloring, and glitter.

Raw Ingredients:

110 g sodium bicarbonate
55 g citric acid
55 g arrowroot powder
40 g dead sea mineral salt (ultra-fine)
20 g pink Himalayan salt
1/2 tsp white kaolin clay
1/2 tsp cocoa powder extract
15 ml safflower oil
10 ml witch hazel water (put in a spray bottle)
1.25 ml natural preservative (i.e., Leucidal® Liquid Complete)
10–15 drops of vanilla essential oil

Kitchen Tools:

You will need a bowl, measuring spoons, scale, gloves, spray bottle, and a medium-sized metal bath bomb mold.

Recipe Prep Time

Prep Time: 20 minutes
Set Time: 30 minutes
Qty: 2 bath bombs

Method:

1. In a large bowl, combine all dry ingredients-sodium bicarbonate, citric acid, arrowroot powder, pink himalayan salt, dead sea salt-ultra fine, clay and botanical extract.
2. Wearing gloves, mix well with your hands making sure the mixture is clump free.
3. Add in the safflower oil, essential oils and preservative.
4. While mixing with your hands, spritz witch hazel into the mixture. Continue to spritz until the mixture holds together without crumbling.
5. Loosely pack the mixture into one half of the metal bath bomb mold; repeat the process for other half.
6. Firmly press the two packed molds together. Press and hold for about 30 seconds. Tap on the metal mold with a spoon (this helps to gently release the mixture).
7. You can pop the bath bomb in the fridge for 30 minutes or leave out overnight at room temperature to fully harden.

Coconut-Pomegranate Mineral Body Scrub

Exfoliate, hydrate, and replenish lost minerals with our famously fresh coconut-pomegranate body scrub.

Raw Ingredients:

500 g dead sea mineral salt (ultra-fine, not too coarse)
30 ml jojoba cold-pressed carrier oil
40 g extra virgin organic coconut oil
1/2 tsp pomegranate powder extract
20 drops of your favorite essential oil

Kitchen Tools:

You will need a large bowl, scale, spatula, measuring spoon, and a jar.

Recipe Prep Time

Prep Time: 10 minutes
Set Time: 10 minutes
Qty: 500 g jar

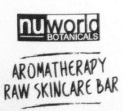

Method:

1. Pour mineral salt into a clean bowl.
2. Add in the extra virgin organic coconut oil.
3. "Wet" the salt-balm with the carrier oil.
4. Sprinkle in the raw powder extract.
5. Add in the essential oil.
6. Mix all ingredients together.
7. Hand pack in a 500g container.

Vegan Detox Deodorant

Our waterless, chemical-free deodorant recipe works to detox your pores and absorb odor while nourishing your sensitive skin with gentle plant oils.

Raw Ingredients:

15 raw shea butter
3 g raw mango butter
3 g extra virgin organic coconut oil
3 g carnauba wax
2.5 g arrowroot powder
1.25 g bentonite clay
6–8 drops essential oils

Kitchen Tools:

You will need a double boiler, scale, small pot, whisk, spatula, measuring spoons, beaker, and a jar.

Recipe Prep Time
Prep Time: 15 minutes
Set Time: 20 minutes
Qty: 30 g jar

Method:

1. In a double boiler, gradually melt raw shea butter, raw mango butter, extra virgin coconut oil, and carnauba wax.
2. Transfer to a beaker and then add in the arrowroot powder and bentonite clay.
3. Whisk fast as the mixture solidifies quickly.
4. Add in the essential oils.
5. Whisk again then pour the mixture into your jar.
6. Pop in the fridge cap off for about 20 minutes.

3-in-1 Body, Bath & Hair Oil

Our top-selling 3-in-1 Aromatherapy oil. This anxiety-relieving blend is ultra-calming, super-hydrating, and multi-tasking. Use on body to moisturize, hair to tame frizz, or add a few drops to your bathwater. Don't forget to breathe in the transforming aroma.

Raw Ingredients:

60% sweet almond oil
30% jojoba oil
5 drops pomegranate oil
5 drops meadowfoam oil
5–7 drops rosehip oil
8 drops lavender essential oil
6 drops sweet orange essential oil
4 drops rosewood essential oil
2 drops ylang-ylang essential oil
1 drop vitamin E
1–2 drops sea buckthorn oil

Kitchen Tools:

You will need a small funnel and bottle.

Prep Time: 8 minutes
Set Time: 5 minutes
Qty: 50 ml bottle

Method:

1. In a bottle, add your carrier oils—pomegranate, rosehip, and meadowfoam.
2. Add in essential oils—rosewood, lavender, ylang-ylang, and sweet orange.
3. Add in base carrier oils—cold-pressed jojoba and sweet almond oil.
4. Add in the vitamin E.
5. Add in the sea buckthorn oil.
6. Put the cap on and shake well.

Tamanu-Turmeric Healing Balm

All-natural antibacterial spot treatment for acne, eczema, skin rashes, scars, and more!

Raw Ingredients:

45 g raw tamanu butter
4 g carnauba wax
1/2 tsp extra virgin organic coconut oil
1.25 ml safflower oil
1.25 ml calendula oil
1/4 tsp turmeric powder extract
2 drops sea buckthorn oil
6–8 drops tea tree essential oil
1 drop vitamin E

Kitchen Tools:

You will need a double boiler, small pot, scale, whisk, spatula, measuring spoons, beaker, and a jar.

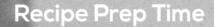

Recipe Prep Time

Prep Time: 15 minutes
Set Time: 20 minutes
Qty: 60 g jar

Method:

1. In a double boiler, gradually melt raw tamanu butter, extra virgin organic coconut oil, and carnauba wax.
2. Mix in safflower oil and calendula oil.
3. Once melted, add in turmeric powder and stir well.
4. Transfer into a beaker or Pyrex; add in sea buckthorn oil, tea tree essential oil, and vitamin E.
5. Whisk fast as the mixture solidifies quickly.
6. Pour into the empty container.
7. Pop in the fridge (cap on) for about 20 minutes to set faster.
8. Allow to solidify thoroughly before using.

Blue Chamomile Eczema-Relief Balm

A powerful anti-inflammatory balm that helps soothe and calm dry, itchy, and irritated skin conditions like psoriasis and eczema.

Raw Ingredients:

115 g aloe butter
10 drops calendula oil
15 drops blue chamomile essential oil
2 drops vitamin E

Kitchen Tools:

You will need a double boiler, small pot, scale, spatula, whisk, beaker, and a jar.

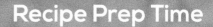

Prep Time: 5 minutes
Set Time: 20 minutes
Qty: 120 g jar

Method:

1. In a double boiler, gradually melt raw aloe butter.
2. Once melted, add in calendula oil and stir well.
3. Transfer into beaker or Pyrex; add in blue chamomile essential oil and vitamin E. Mix well.
4. Pour into the empty container.
5. Pop in the fridge (cap on) for about 20 minutes to set faster.

Artisan Donut Cleansing Bar

Our artisan clay bar is known for deep-cleansing the skin and drawing out impurities without drying the skin. Looks just like a gourmet baked treat (but please do not eat)!

Raw Ingredients:

70 g shea melt & pour soap base
20 g shea melt & pour base (for drizzle icing)
1/8 tsp French green clay
1/8 tsp spirulina powder extract
1/8 tsp loofah
10 drops lime essential oil

Kitchen Tools:

You will need a double boiler, small pot, scale, beaker, whisk, spatula, measuring spoons, squeeze bottle, and a donut-shaped silicone mold.

thod:

In a double boiler, gradually melt soap
base.
Once melted, transfer into a beaker.
Mix in the powder extract, clay, and
exfoliant.
Add in essential oils.
Pour the liquid into the mold.
Carefully transfer the molds to the
fridge for about 20–25 minutes to set
faster.
Once the bars have solidified, remove it
from the silicone mold.

zzle Icing:

In a separate pot, melt down 20g shea
soap base.
Once melted, transfer it into a squeeze
bottle.
Working quickly, drizzle on top of your
donut cleansing bar.
Allow bar to solidify thoroughly before
using.

Sports Mineral Bath Soak

Our best-selling bath soak has over 84 trace minerals to help soothe sore, achy muscles and joints, post-workout. Also helpful for relieving arthritis and eczema.

Raw Ingredients:

100 g pink Himalayan salt
150 g Dead Sea mineral salt
8 drops cold-pressed argan oil
1 drop vitamin E
5 drops wintergreen essential oil
5 drops eucalyptus essential oil
5 drops peppermint essential oil
1/2 tsp seaweed powder extract (or your choice extract)

Kitchen Tools:

You will need a bowl, spatula, dropper, scale, measuring spoon, and a jar.

Method:

1. Pour pink himalayan salt and dead sea mineral salt into your bowl.
2. Add in the argan oil and vitamin e.
3. Add in the essential oils–wintergreen, eucalyptus, peppermint.
4. Add in the seaweed powder extract.
5. Mix well.
6. Transfer mixture into the jar.

Waterless Lemon-Shea Body Butter

Yes, you can make a body butter without the use of water! Our waterless body butter is vegan and 100% naturally active.

Raw Ingredients:

---

25 g raw shea butter
12 g extra virgin organic coconut oil
6 ml sweet almond oil
6 ml safflower oil
3 ml jojoba oil
2 g carnauba wax
8 drops lemon essential oil
2 drops grapefruit essential oil
1–2 drops vitamin E

Kitchen Tools:

You will need a double boiler, small pot, scale, whisk, spatula, measuring spoons, beaker, and a jar.

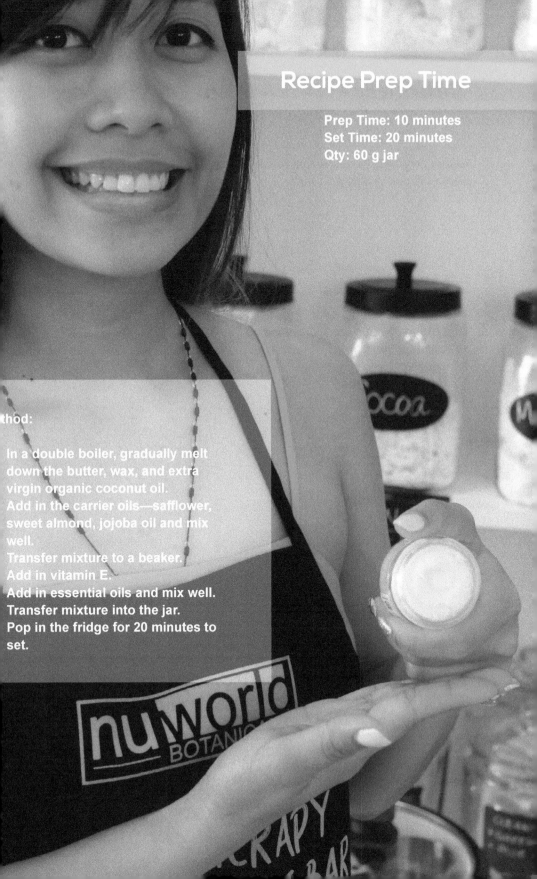

Recipe Prep Time

Prep Time: 10 minutes
Set Time: 20 minutes
Qty: 60 g jar

Method:

In a double boiler, gradually melt down the butter, wax, and extra virgin organic coconut oil.
Add in the carrier oils—safflower, sweet almond, jojoba oil and mix well.
Transfer mixture to a beaker.
Add in vitamin E.
Add in essential oils and mix well.
Transfer mixture into the jar.
Pop in the fridge for 20 minutes to set.

Orange Butter & Apricot Foot Scrub Bar

Glides on and sinks in with a touch of exfoliation—this solid bar is perfect for dry heels and feet.

Raw Ingredients:

25 g Dead Sea mineral salt (ultra-fine)
20 g orange butter
10 ml grape seed oil
6 g candelilla wax
1/2 tsp apricot shells
6–8 drops essential oil
2 drops vitamin E

Kitchen Tools:

You will need a double boiler, small pot, scale, beaker, whisk, spatula, measuring spoons, and silicone molds.

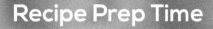

Recipe Prep Time

Prep Time: 15 minutes
Set Time: 30 minutes
Qty: 2 x 30 g bar

Method:

1. In a double boiler, gradually melt down the butter and wax.
2. Mix in grape seed oil. Stir well.
3. Once melted, pour the mixture into a clean beaker or Pyrex and add in dead sea salt, apricot shells, vitamin E, and essential oil. Mix well.
4. Transfer into the mold.
5. Pop in the fridge for 30 minutes or until solid.

Natural Perfume Roll-On

An aromatic blend of pure and exotic essential oils creates a subtle all-natural perfume.

Raw Ingredients:

6 ml of safflower oil
2 ml of jojoba oil
5 drops jasmine essential oil
5 drops ylang-ylang essential oil
3 drops rose essential oil
2 drops sandalwood essential oil
1 drop vitamin E

Kitchen Tools:

You will need a measuring spoon, funnel, and roll-on bottle.

Recipe Prep Time

Recipe Prep Time
Prep Time: 5 minutes
Set Time: 5 minutes
Qty: 10 ml roll-on

Method:

1. Fill the roll-on bottle about 85% with jojoba and safflower oil (leave room for your essential oils and to pop the roller ball back in).
2. Add in essential oils.
3. Add in vitamin E.
4. Pop the roller ball back in and cap.
5. Shake bottle and roll on wrists/back of ears.

Raw Skincare

Recipes

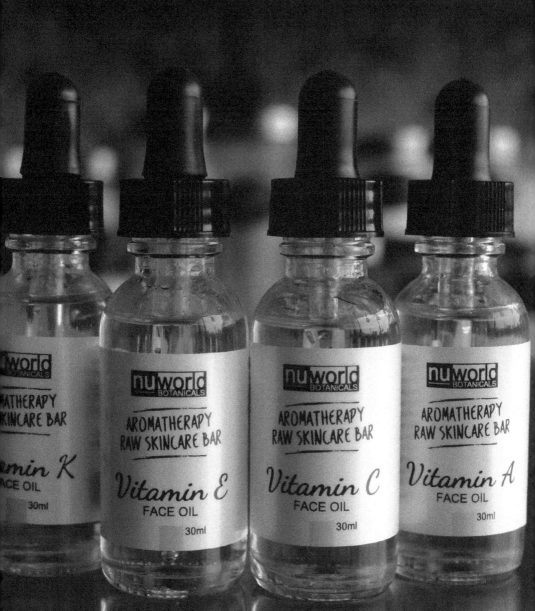

Creamy Mango-Apricot Exfoliator

Creamy but with some scrub in it. This recipe works well for drier skin types.

Raw Ingredients:

70 g creamy vegan base butter*
1/4 tsp mango powder extract
1/4 tsp apricot shells
1 tsp carrier oil (i.e., jojoba oil)
10 drops essential oil (i.e., lemon, rose)

*Try our vegan butter base or make your own from scratch. See our **recipe** *Whipped Rosehip–Strawberry Body Butter.*

Kitchen Tools:

You will need a double boiler, small pot, scale, whisk, spatula, measuring spoons, beaker, and a jar.

Recipe Prep Time

Prep Time: 10 minutes
Set Time: 15 minutes
Qty: 60 g jar

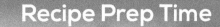

Method:

1. In a double boiler, gently melt down the cream base to a semi-liquid state.
2. Add in the mango extract and whisk until blended.
3. Add in the carrier oil.
4. Add in the exfoliator—apricot shells—and whisk until combined.
5. Transfer the liquid cream into a beaker and add in the essential oils.
6. Pop in the fridge for about 15 minutes to set faster or leave out for 30 minutes at room temperature to thicken.
7. Transfer mixture into the jar.

Simple Cleansing Oil + Makeup Remover

The "oil cleansing method" uses natural oils to cleanse the skin gently and balance the skin's natural oils. Works nicely to remove makeup too.

To Use: Warm a small amount of oil in the palm of your hands. Gently massage into dry skin and smooth over eyes. Use circular massage movements to stimulate the skin, dislodge dead skin cells, and lift away impurities and make-up. Wash away with our warmed cotton-organic muslin cloth (create a steam facial).

Raw Ingredients:

50% jojoba oil
50% apricot kernel oil
1 drop vitamin E

Kitchen Tools:

You will need a funnel and a bottle

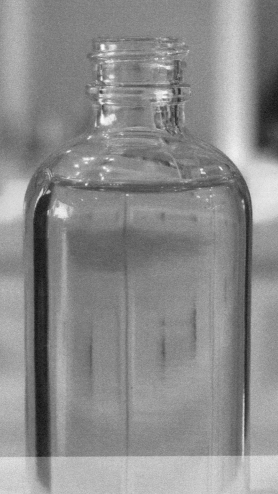

Prep Time: 5 minutes
Set Time: 5 minutes
Qty: 60 ml bottle

Method:

1. **Fill bottle 50% with jojoba oil.**
2. **Fill bottle 50% with apricot kernel oil.**
3. **Add in vitamin E.**
4. **Put cap on and shake well.**

Blue Tansy + Honey Whipped Face Butter

Our antibacterial, anti-inflammatory face butter cream is super light-weight and perfect for sensitive, irritated, or problematic skin. This includes acne-prone skin and eczema.

Raw Ingredients:

70 g creamy vegan base butter*
5 drops apricot kernel oil
5 drops carrot oil
5 drops pomegranate oil
1/4 tsp honey powder extract
1 drop sea buckthorn oil
1 drop blue tansy essential oil
1 drop vitamin E

*Try our vegan butter base or make your own from scratch. See our recipe *Whipped Rosehip–Strawberry Body Butter*.

Kitchen Tools:

You will need a double boiler, small pot, scale, whisk, spatula, measuring spoons, beaker, and a jar.

Prep Time: 10 minutes
Set Time: 15 minutes
Qty: 60 g jar

Method:

1. In a double boiler, gently melt down the cream base to a semi-liquid state.
2. Add in the carrier oils.
3. Add in the powder extract and whisk until combined.
4. Transfer the liquid cream into a beaker, add in vitamin E, essential oil, and sea buckthorn oil.
5. Pop in the fridge for about 15 minutes to set faster or leave out at room temperature to thicken.
6. Transfer mixture into the jar.

Matcha-Honey Exfoliating Facial Bar

This natural soap bar is 100% natural and SLS-free. Use on the face to cleanse and exfoliate. Matcha can help reduce the redness associated with rosacea and even acne, while honey delivers antibacterial properties.

Raw Ingredients:

140 g honey melt & pour soap base
1/4 tsp French green clay
1/4 tsp matcha green tea powder extract
1/4 tsp ground loofah
10–20 drops essential oils (optional)

Kitchen Tools:

You will need a double boiler, small pot, scale, beakers, whisk, spatula, measuring spoons, and silicone molds.

Prep Time: 15 minutes
Set Time: 25 minutes
Qty: 2 x 70 g bar

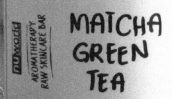

Method:

1. In a double boiler, gradually melt the soap base.
2. Once melted, mix in the matcha green tea powder extract, green clay and loofah. Stir well.
3. Transfer into a beaker or Pyrex and add in essential oils.
4. Quickly pour the liquid evenly into the mold.
5. Sprinkle remaining loofah on top of each one (optional).
6. Carefully transfer the molds to the fridge for about 20-25 minutes to set faster.
7. Once the bars have solidified, remove the soaps from silico molds.

To make layers: At step 2, leave out the matcha green tea powder extract and green clay. Fill molds half way. Add the matcha green tea powder, essential oil and green clay to the leftover mixture in the beaker, mix and pour into mold as the second layer. Proceed to step 5.

Blue Tansy-Aloe Soothing Cleansing Bar

Our most calming cleansing bar ever pairs soothing Aloe vera with our powerhouse anti-inflammatory blue tansy essential oil. Calms down inflamed, red, and irritated skin.

Raw Ingredients:

70 g aloe vera melt & pour soap base
1/4 tsp jojoba beads
1/4 tsp banana powder extract
1/4 tsp kaolin white clay
2 drops blue tansy essential oil
8 drops rosewood essential oil

Kitchen Tools:

You will need a double boiler, small pot, scale, beakers, whisk, spatula, measuring spoons, and silicone molds.

Prep Time: 15 minutes
Set Time: 25 minutes
Qty: 70 g bar

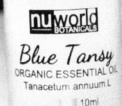

nuworld
BOTANICALS

Blue Tansy
ORGANIC ESSENTIAL OIL
Tanacetum annuum L

10ml

Method:

1. In a double boiler, gradually melt the soap base.
2. Once melted, mix in the jojoba beads, clay and powder extract.
3. Transfer into a beaker and add in essential oils.
4. Quickly pour the liquid evenly into the mold.
5. Carefully transfer the molds to the fridge for about
   20-25 minutes to set faster.
6. Once the bars have solidified, remove from silicone mold.

To make layers: At step 2, leave out the banana powder
extract and kaolin white clay. Fill molds half way. Add the banana
powder extract, essential oil and kaolin white clay to the leftover
mixture in the beaker, mix and pour into mold as the second layer.
Proceed to step 5.

Raw Fruit Powder Face Exfoliator

100% raw and concentrated fruit exfoliator. Rich in natural vitamins, antioxidants, and raw exfoliants.

To Use: Pour a 1/4 size amount of powder into your hands and slowly add water, mix to a paste. Using gentle circular motions, massage onto your face for about one minute then rinse well with warm water.

Raw Ingredients:

80% kaolin white clay
1 tsp fig seeds (ground powder) or any raw exfoliant
1/4 tsp strawberry powder extract
1/4 tsp mango powder extract
1/4 tsp pineapple powder extract
1/8 tsp matcha green tea powder extract

Kitchen Tools:

You will need measuring spoons and a jar.

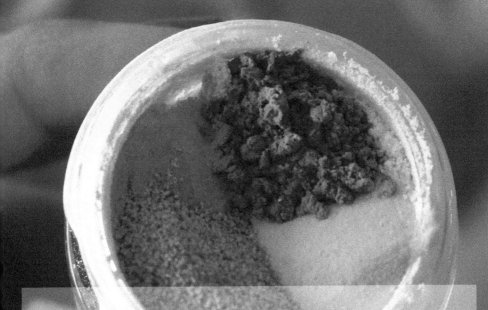

Recipe Prep Time

Prep Time: 5 minutes
Set Time: 5 minutes
Qty: 30 g jar

Method:

1. Fill jar 80% full with kaolin white clay.
2. Add in the powder extracts and raw exfoliant.
3. Add in the super-booster matcha powder.
4. Top up with more kaolin white clay until jar is full.
5. Shake well and it's ready to use.

5-Minute Mineral Clay Mask

Our signature clay mask is a powdered, ready-to-mix mask that purifies the skin while targeting specific skin conditions.
Choose the extracts and clays that are right for you!

To Use: Mix 1 tsp of clay with about 1 tsp of water to form a thin paste. Apply a thin layer to your face (avoiding eyes) for five minutes then rinse.

Raw Ingredients:

40% Moroccan rhassoul clay
40% French pink clay
1 tsp kaolin white clay
1/4 tsp wasabi powder extract
1/4 tsp matcha green tea powder extract
1/4 tsp turmeric powder extract
1/8 tsp aloe vera powder extract

Kitchen Tools:

You will need measuring spoons and a jar.

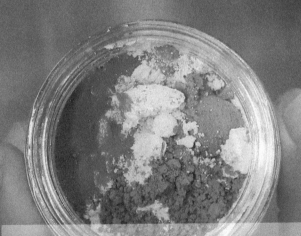

Method:

1. Add about 40% rhassoul clay and about 40% pink clay to your jar.
2. Add in your kaolin white clay.
3. Add in your extracts.
4. Top up with more clay until jar is full.
5. Shake well and combine before use.

Chocolate-Fennel Vitamin Cleansing Bar

This natural soap bar is 100% natural and SLS-free. Use on the face to cleanse, repair, and protect skin from free radicals. Fennel is an excellent source of vitamin C essential to collagen production. The antioxidants present in cocoa boost the elasticity of your skin.

Raw Ingredients:

140 g shea melt & pour soap base
1/4 tsp kaolin white clay
1/4 tsp cocoa powder extract
1/4 tsp ground loofah
10–20 drops sweet fennel essential oil

Kitchen Tools:

You will need a double boiler, small pot, scale, beaker, whisk, spatula, measuring spoons, and silicone molds.

Method:

1. In a double boiler, gradually melt the soap base.
2. Once melted, mix in the kaolin white clay, cocoa powder extract and loofah. Stir well.
3. Transfer into a beaker or Pyrex, add in essential oils.
4. Then quickly pour the liquid evenly into the mold.
5. Sprinkle remaining loofah on top of each one (optional).
6. Carefully transfer the molds to the fridge for about 20-25 minutes to set faster.
7. Once the bars have solidified, remove from silicone molds.
8. Allow your cleansing bar to solidify thoroughly before using.

To make layers: At step 2, leave out the cocoa powder extract and kaolin white clay. Fill molds half way. Add the cocoa powder extract, essential oil and kaolin white clay to the leftover mixture in the beaker, mix and pour into mold as the second layer. Proceed to step 5.

Hydrate + Exfoliate Lip Balms- Set of Four

Create 3 hydrating balms and 1 exfoliating lip balm with this one recipe. Watermelon extract is rich in vitamin C and natural alpha-hydroxy acids and creates a natural exfoliating lip balm.

Raw Ingredients:

18 g shea butter
2 g cocoa butter
2 g extra virgin organic coconut oil
3 g candelilla wax
5 ml oil blend (i.e. olive + hemp seed)
1 drop vitamin E
1/8 tsp watermelon powder extract
4–6 drops essential oils (per tube)

Kitchen Tools:

You will need a double boiler, scale, small pot, whisk, spatula, measuring spoons, beaker, and four lip balm containers.

Method:

1. In a double boiler, combine and gradually melt the raw shea butter, cocoa butter, extra virgin coconut oil and candelilla wax.
2. Mix in the oil blend (olive oil, hemp seed oil and vitamin e).
3. Once melted, remove from heat and transfer to a clean beaker.
4. At this point, you could add in your favorite essential oils or you could dispense the oil drops into each individual lip balm tube to create different scents.
5. Working quickly before it solidifies, pour the liquid mixture into the 3 lip balm tubes. These are your hydrating lip balms.
6. In the remaining mixture in the beaker, add in the watermelon extract.
7. Mix quickly, then pour the liquid into the last lip balm tube- this is your exfoliating lip balm.
8. Pop in the fridge for 15 minutes to set faster.
9. Allow your lip balm to solidify thoroughly before using.

Carrot Melting Cleansing Balm

Our best-selling cleansing balm cleanses and removes make-up while improving skin tone, clarity, and smoothness. Carrot butter is rich in beta-carotene (a form of vitamin A), perfect for very dry skin types.

To Use: Warm a small amount of carrot balm in the palm of your hands. Gently massage into dry skin and smooth over eyes (also removes make-up). Use circular massage movements to stimulate the skin, dislodge dead skin cells, and lift away impurities and make-up. Wash away with our warmed cotton-organic warmed muslin cloth (create a steam facial). Use a touch of balm as your daily under-eye treatment.

Raw Ingredients:

50 g raw carrot butter
1 tsp extra virgin organic coconut oil
1.5 ml apricot kernel oil
1.5 ml jojoba oil
1.5 ml meadowfoam oil
1 drop sea buckthorn oil
1 drop vitamin E

Kitchen Tools:

You will need a double boiler, small pot, scale, whisk, spatula, measuring spoons, beaker, and a jar.

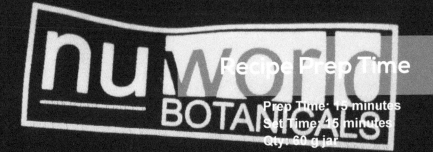

AROMATHERAPY
RAW SKINCARE BAR

Method:

1. In a double boiler, gently melt the raw carrot butter, extra virgin organic coconut oil, and whisk until melted.
2. Once melted, remove from heat.
3. Add in the jojoba oil, apricot oil, meadowfoam oil, and stir.
4. Transfer to a beaker or Pyrex.
5. Add in the sea buckthorn and vitamin E. Whisk.
6. Pour the mixture into a jar (lid on tightly).
7. Pop the jar in the fridge for about 10–15 minutes, to set faster.

Vitamin C Facial Oil

Moisturize, brighten, and protect the skin from daily free radical damage with nature's richest source of vitamin C—Sea Buckthorn. Use daily on clean fresh skin and under make-up as a primer and daily moisturizer.

Raw Ingredients:

60% jojoba oil
30% safflower oil
5 drops borage oil
5 drops meadowfoam oil
5 drops rosehip oil
3 drops sea buckthorn oil
1 drop vitamin E

Kitchen Tools:

You will need a dropper, beaker, and a bottle

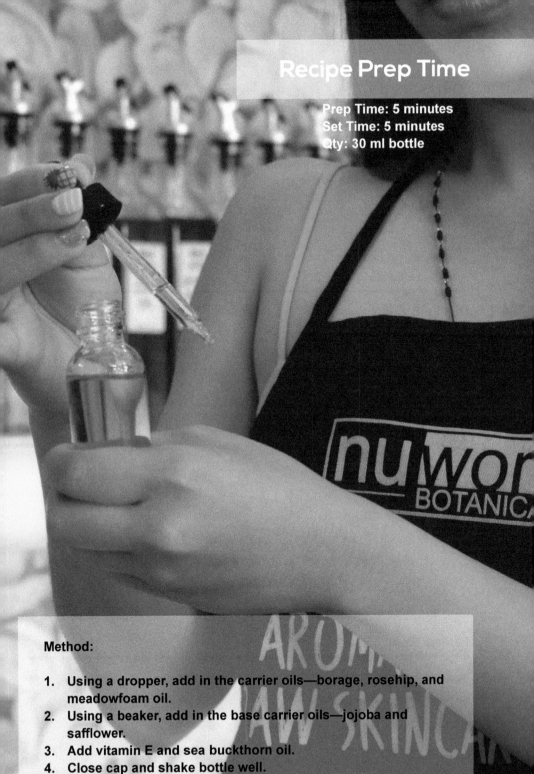

Prep Time: 5 minutes
Set Time: 5 minutes
Qty: 30 ml bottle

Method:

1. **Using a dropper, add in the carrier oils—borage, rosehip, and meadowfoam oil.**
2. **Using a beaker, add in the base carrier oils—jojoba and safflower.**
3. **Add vitamin E and sea buckthorn oil.**
4. **Close cap and shake bottle well.**

Mineral Clay Mask Facial Bar

Our famous powdered clay mask gets transformed into a travel-sized solid bar. Quick and easy to use on the fly, just wet the bar and apply to damp skin.

Raw Ingredients:

50 g French pink clay
30 g kaolin white clay
15 ml aloe vera juice
15 ml witch hazel water
4 g raw shea butter
1.25 ml natural preservative (i.e., Leucidal® Liquid Complete)
1 drop vitamin E

Kitchen Tools:

You will need a double boiler, small pot, scale, bowl, whisk, gloves, parchment paper, and silicone molds.

Recipe Prep Time

Prep Time: 10 minutes
Set Time: 20 minutes
Qty: 2 x 30 g bar

Method:

1. In a double boiler, gently melt down the shea butter.
2. In a separate bowl, add in the clays and whisk. Add in the Aloe vera and witch hazel and mix with your hands (gloves on).
3. Transfer the melted shea to the beaker.
4. Add in vitamin E and the natural preservative to the beaker.
5. Pour the shea mixture into the clay bowl.
6. Using your hands (with gloves) combine all ingredients until it's packed.
7. Pack and press the mixture well into your molds (molds can be lined with parchment paper for better release).
8. Pop in the fridge for 20 minutes to set faster.

Mango Melting Eye Balm

An upgrade to an eye cream! This luxe eye balm is rich in vitamin K and helps with under-eye dark circles.

Raw Ingredients:

20 g raw mango butter
30 g raw carrot butter
1/2 tsp extra virgin organic coconut oil
1/2 tsp apricot kernel oil
1/2 tsp meadowfoam oil
2 drops sea buckthorn oil
1 drop vitamin E

Kitchen Tools:

You will need a double boiler, small pot, scale, whisk, spatula, measuring spoons, beaker, and a jar.

e: 15 mi
: 20 min
0 g jars

NGO

ER

Method:

1. In a double boiler, gently melt down the butters and coconut oil.
2. Add in the carrier oils.
3. Mix well, then transfer to a beaker.
4. Add in the sea buckthorn and vitamin E.
5. Whisk well until combined.
6. Pour into your jar.
7. Pop in the fridge for 20 minutes to set faster.

Raw Haircare Recipes

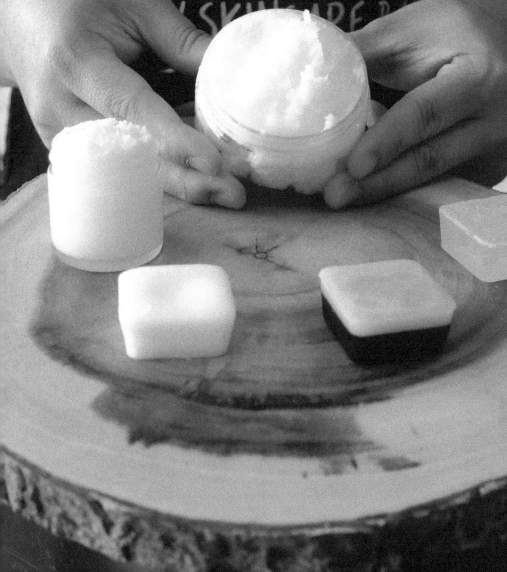

Charcoal Scalp Detox Bar

Use this bar on wet hair before you shampoo to help lift dead skin cells and oil off the scalp. Made with loofah to help cut through any stubborn buildup, as well.

To use: Wet your hair and the bar. Massage the bar onto your scalp. Put the bar down and work in the product with your fingers. Rinse, then shampoo and condition.

Raw Ingredients:

140 g honey melt & pour soap base
1/4 tsp kaolin white clay
1/4 tsp activated bamboo charcoal
1/4 tsp ground loofah
10–20 drops essential oils

Kitchen Tools:

You will need a double boiler, small pot, scale, beaker, whisk, spatula, measuring spoons, and silicone molds.

Prep Time: 15 minutes
Set Time: 25 minutes
Qty: 2 x 70 g bar

Method:

1. In a double boiler, gradually melt the soap base.
2. Once melted, mix in the kaolin white clay, activated bamboo charcoal and loofah. Stir well.
3. Transfer into a beaker or Pyrex and add in the essential oils.
4. Quickly pour the liquid evenly into the mold.
5. Sprinkle remaining loofah on top of each one (optional).
6. Carefully transfer the molds to the fridge for about 25 minutes to set faster.
7. Once the bars have solidified, remove from silicone molds.
8. Allow your cleansing bar to solidify thoroughly before using.

To make layers: At step 2 , leave out the charcoal and fill molds half way. Add the charcoal and essential oil to the leftover mixture in the beaker, mix and pour into mold as the second layer. Proceed to step 5.

Argan-Rosemary Vitamin Shampoo Bar

Cleanse your scalp while nourishing your strands with this zero-waste solid shampoo bar. Perfect for travel.

To use: Wet your hair and the bar. Slide the bar from root to tip a few times. Put the bar down and work in the product with your fingers. Rinse and follow with our conditioner bar.

Raw Ingredients:

140 g argan melt & pour soap base
5 ml castor oil and vegetable glycerin combined (half/half)
5 ml olive oil
20 drops of rosemary essential oil

Kitchen Tools:

You will need a double boiler, small pot, beaker, spatula, whisk, and silicone molds.

Recipe Prep Time

Prep Time: 15 minutes
Set Time: 20 minutes
Qty: 2 x 70 g bar

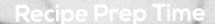

Method:

1. In a double boiler, gradually melt the argan soap base.
2. Once melted, pour into a beaker or Pyrex.
3. Add in the oils and mix.
4. Working quickly, pour evenly into the silicone soap molds.
5. Pop in the fridge for about 20 minutes to set faster.
6. Remove from molds and use. Allow your shampoo bar to solidify thoroughly before using.

Murumuru Hair Butter

Our super popular Murumuru hair butter—strengthens and repairs dry, brittle, and damaged hair.

To Use: On damp or dry hair, massage a quarter-sized amount on the scalp and move another quarter-sized through your hair strands to the end. Massage the entire head to ensure even distribution. Comb through hair. Leave in for 30 minutes or preferably overnight then shampoo, condition, style as usual. Use twice a week.

Raw Ingredients:

5 g murumuru butter
5 g tucuma butter
35 g raw mango butter
20 ml argan oil
1 tbsp marula oil
1 tbsp extra virgin organic coconut oil (heaping)
2 drops vitamin E

Kitchen Tools:

You will need a double boiler, metal pots, electric whisk, spatula, scale, measuring spoons, beaker, and a jar.

Prep Time: 20 minutes
Set Time: 30 minutes
Qty: 120 g jar

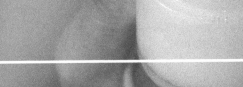

Method:

1. In a double boiler, gradually melt the murumuru butter, mango butter and tucuma butter.
2. Mix in the argan oil, marula oil and extra virgin organic coconut oil.
3. Once melted, pour mixture into a clean beaker or Pyrex and add in the vitamin e. Mix well.
4. Pop in fridge for about 30 minutes or until semi-solid.
5. Using an electric hand mixer, whisk for about 3 minutes or until creamy.
6. Scoop into jar.

Murumuru Hair Conditioner Bar

This bar restores hair health, treating dry and damaged hair with intense moisture. Improves hair flexibility and strength, protecting against split ends and other damage.

To Use: After shampooing, slide the bar over the ends of your hair, then into the scalp. Put the bar down and massage the conditioner into your scalp and hair. Rinse and you're good to go!

Raw Ingredients:

---

15 g raw murumuru butter
50 g emulsifying wax
5 ml argan oil
5 ml apricot kernel oil
2.5 ml vegetable glycerin
15 ml witch hazel water
2.5 ml natural preservative (i.e., Leucidal® Liquid Complete)
15 drops total essential oil (i.e., lemon, lime)
1 drop vitamin E

Kitchen Tools:

You will need a double boiler, metal pot, whisk, spatula, measuring spoons, beaker, and silicone molds.

Method:

1. In a double boiler, gradually melt the murumuru butter and emulsifying wax.
2. Once melted, add in the oils—argan, apricot kernel and the vegetable glycerin.
3. Add in the witch hazel and continually whisk until combined (about 1-2 minutes).
4. Transfer into beaker or Pyrex. Add in your essential oil, natural preservative and vitamin e.
5. Whisk and work quickly as the mixture solidifies quickly.
6. Pour into your molds.
7. Pop in the fridge for about 15-20 minutes to set faster.
8. Allow your bars to solidify thoroughly before using.

Coconut-Banana Nourishing Hair Mask

No matter what your hair type is, all strands are deserving of nourishment with this high dosage of vitamins and nutrients.

Raw Ingredients:

120 g extra virgin organic coconut oil
6–8 drops marula oil
3 drops macadamia oil
3 drops argan oil
3 drops avocado oil
1/4 tsp banana powder extract
8–10 drops essential oil

Kitchen Tools:

You will need a whisk, spatula, and a jar.

Recipe Prep Time

Method:

1. Fill jar with our extra virgin organic coconut oil.
2. Add in marula oil, macadamia oil, argan oil, and avocado oil.
3. Add in the powder extract.
4. Add in the essential oils.
5. Mix well.

Blue Tansy-Marula Soothing Scalp Oil

Soothe and treat a dry, itchy, and flaky scalp with nature's power anti-inflammatory blue tansy and marula's emollient and moisturizing benefits.

To Use: On damp hair, place the dropper on the scalp at the hair root (in sections) and move through your scalp to disperse the oil. Massage the entire head to ensure even distribution. Comb through hair. Leave in for 30 minutes or overnight then shampoo, condition, style as usual. Use at least twice a week.

Raw Ingredients:

20 ml olive oil
5 ml macadamia nut oil
5 ml marula oil
3 drops blue tansy essential oil
1 drop vitamin E

Kitchen Tools:

You will need a small funnel, measuring spoons, and a bottle.

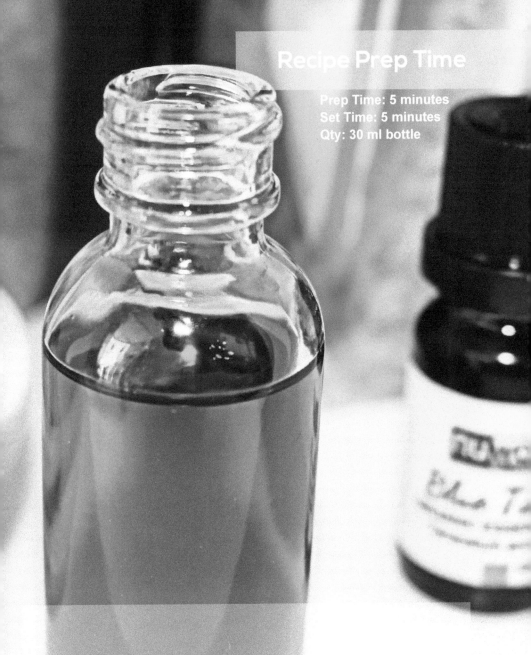

Method:

1. Fill bottle 90% with cold-pressed carrier oils.
2. Add in essential oil.
3. Add in vitamin E.
4. Close cap and shake bottle well before use.

Raw Makeup Recipes

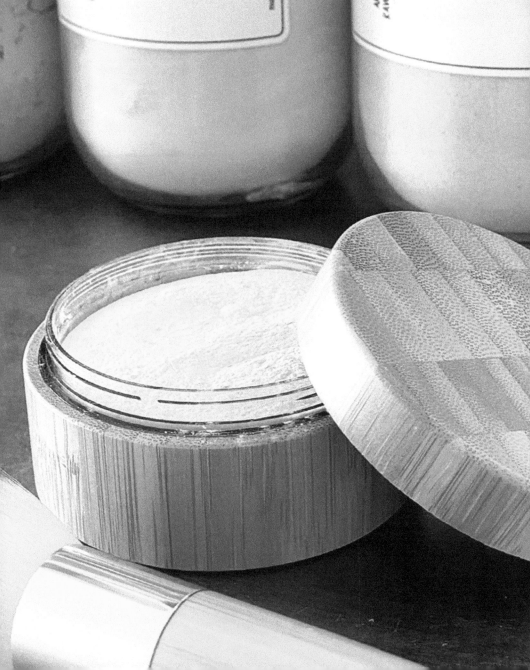

Blue Lavender Eye Shadow

Packed with skin-nourishing vitamins, this naturally pressed powder eye-shadow blends smoothly and effortlessly.

Raw Ingredients:

4 drops vegetable glycerin
2 drops meadowfoam oil
2 drops raspberry oil
3 drops aloe vera oil
1/8 tsp silver mineral mica powder
1/2 tsp turquoise natural mineral pigment
1/4 tsp blue lavender natural mineral pigment

Kitchen Tools:

You will need a small bowl, measuring spoons, wax paper, flat utensil, dropper, and a jar.

Recipe Prep Time

Prep Time: 5 minutes
Set Time: 5 minutes
Qty: 3 g jar

Method:

1. In a small bowl, mix the dry micas.
2. Add in the meadowfoam oil, aloe vera oil, raspberry oil, and glycerin.
3. Mix well with a whisk.
4. Transfer into a jar. Press firmly over wax paper using a flat utensil.

Fruit-Mix Cuticle Oil

Brightens nails and exfoliates dead skin cells around cuticles. Treats damaged nails and skin irritation or inflammation around the cuticle.

Raw Ingredients:

4 ml fractionated coconut oil
10 drops fruit mix oil*
6 drops essential oil (optional)

*Our fruit mix oil is a blend of bilberry oil, sugar cane, orange, lemon, and sugar maple.

Kitchen Tools:

You will need a measuring spoon, funnel, and a bottle.

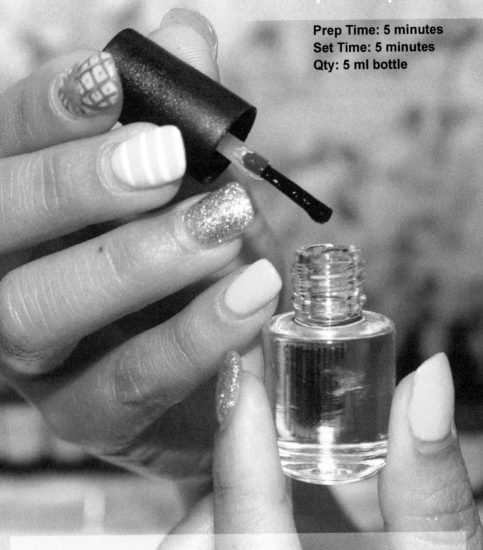

Prep Time: 5 minutes
Set Time: 5 minutes
Qty: 5 ml bottle

Method:

1. With the use of a funnel, add in fractionated coconut oil to the bottle.
2. Add in 10 drops fruit mix oil and essential oil.
3. Close cap and shake bottle well before each use.

Mineral Highlight + Glow Face Oil

Bronze, copper, silver, and gold—mineral micas come in many shades. This nourishing face oil adds an illuminating glow to the high points of your face such as cheekbones, the bridge of the nose, and brow bones.

Raw Ingredients:

80% of jojoba oil
2 drops camellia seed oil
2 drops carrot oil
2 drops meadowfoam oil
2 drops raspberry seed oil
1 tsp natural mineral mica powder (your choice of mica shade)
1 drop vitamin E

Kitchen Tools:

You will need a measuring spoon, dropper, funnel, and a bottle.

Prep Time: 5 minutes
Set Time: 5 minutes
Qty: 30 ml bottle

Method:

1. With the use of a funnel, add the mica powder in the container.
2. Mix in the carrier oils—camellia, carrot, meadowfoam, raspberry, and add the vitamin E.
3. Fill the bottle with jojoba oil.
4. Close cap and shake bottle well before use.

Mineral Glow Cheek Blush

Illuminate your complexion while nourishing your skin with natural vitamins. This lightweight cream blush sinks in and imparts a fresh sheer glow.

Raw Ingredients:

35 g raw carrot butter
2.5 tsp of extra virgin organic coconut oil
1/4 tsp candelilla wax
12 drops jojoba oil
12 drops apricot kernel oil
12 drops meadowfoam oil
1 drop sea buckthorn oil
1/4 tsp silver mica mineral powder
1/4 tsp copper mica mineral powder
1 drop vitamin E

Kitchen Tools:

You will need a double boiler, scale, small pot, whisk, spatula, dropper, measuring spoons, beaker, and jars.

Method:

1. In a double boiler, combine the raw carrot butter, extra virgin organic coconut oil, candelilla wax, and gently whisk until melted.
2. Once melted, turn down heat (or remove from heat).
3. Add in the jojoba oil, apricot kernel oil, and meadowfoam oil.
4. Transfer to a clean beaker. Add in mica powder and mix well.
5. Add in the sea buckthorn oil and vitamin E. Whisk well.
6. Pour the mixture into clean jars and cap tightly.
7. Pop the jar in the fridge for about 10–15 minutes, to set faster.
8. Remove from the fridge and it's ready to use.

Mineral Lip Luminizer

Give your lips a kiss of light and added hydration.

Raw Ingredients:

---

9 ml vegetable glycerin
1.25 ml sunflower oil
15 drops aloe vera oil
15 drops meadowfoam oil
1/2 tsp copper mica (or your choice of mica)
1/2 tsp silver mica (or your choice of mica)
2 drops vitamin E

Kitchen Tools:

You will need a small bowl, whisk, measuring spoons, baking piping bags, and lip tubes.

Prep Time: 10 minutes
Set Time: 10 minutes
Qty: 10 ml tube

Method:

1. In a small bowl, mix in vegetable glycerin and sunflower oil.
2. Add in drops of aloe vera oil and meadowfoam oil.
3. Add in mica powder.
4. Add in vitamin E.
5. Mix well with a whisk.
6. Transfer to the container using piping bags.

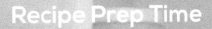

nuworld
BOTANICALS

Murumuru Lash + Brow Boosting Butter

If you wish your lashes were fuller, stronger, and healthier, you'll want to give our lash and brow butter recipe a go!

Raw Ingredients:

---

35 g raw mango butter
5 g murumuru butter
5 g tucuma butter
20 ml argan oil
1 tbsp marula oil
1 tbsp extra virgin organic coconut oil (heaping)
2.5 ml blueberry seed oil
2.5 ml broccoli seed oil
2 drops vitamin E

Kitchen Tools:

You will need a double boiler, metal pot, scale, beaker, measuring spoons, spatula, baking piping bags, electric hand mixer, and lip gloss tubes.

Recipe Prep Time

Prep Time: 15 minutes
Set Time: 30 minutes
Qty: 12 x 10 ml

Method:

1. In a double boiler, gradually melt the murumuru butter, mango butter and tucuma butter.
2. Mix in the argan oil, marula oil, extra virgin organic coconut oil, blueberry oil and broccoli oil.
3. Once melted, pour mixture into a clean beaker or Pyrex and add in vitamin e.
4. Pop in fridge for about 30 minutes or until semi-solid.
5. Using an electric hand mixer, whisk for about 3 minutes or until creamy.
6. Scoop into jar or vials with piping bag.

Superfood Bronzing Setting Powder

Bonus Recipe! A loose bronzing powder that warms up the skin and sets make-up. Made with raw superfood ingredients rich in vitamins A & C. Skin feels silky smooth and looks radiant and glowing.

How to use: Tap a powder brush into the bronzer than sweep it along your cheekbones and around the perimeter of your face, like your temples and forehead—basically all the places where the sun typically hits.

Raw Ingredients:

___

Raw Ingredients:
10 g arrowroot powder
4 g organic coconut powder
1 g organic cocoa powder
2 tsp gold mineral mica powder
1 tsp pearl mineral mica powder
¼ tsp mango extract powder
¼ tsp papaya extract powder
¼ tsp sea buckthorn extract powder
¼ tsp pumpkin extract powder

Kitchen Tools:

___

A scale, bowl and measuring spoons

Prep Time: 5 minutes
Set Time: instant
Qty: 30 g jar

MANGO

PUMPKI

Method:

1. In a mixing bowl add in the arrowroot powder and coconut powder. Mix well together.
2. Add in the superfood extracts and mineral mica powders. Mix well.
3. Using a spoon, transfer the dry powder mixture to your container.

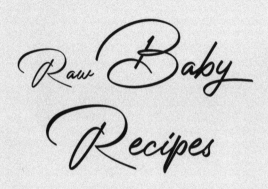

Raw Baby Recipes

Baby recipes with essential oils are intended for children six months of age and older.

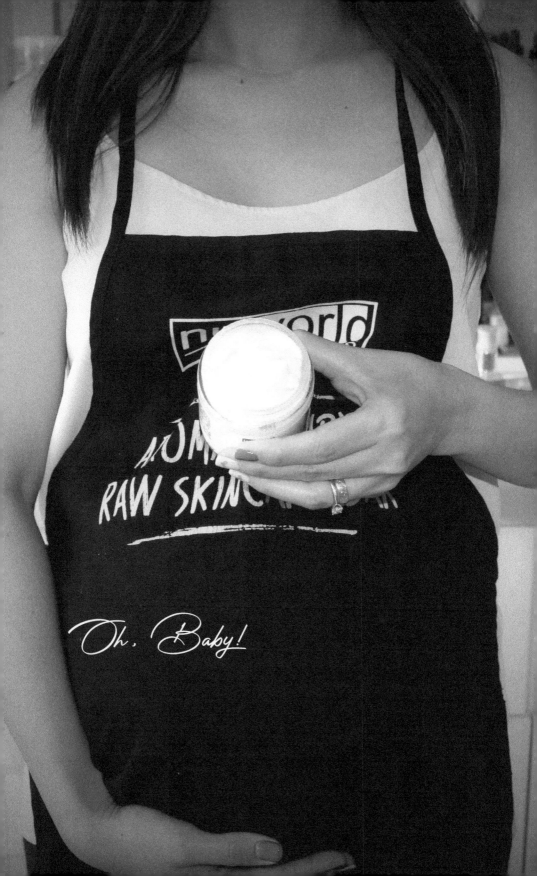

Calendula-Lavender Calming Baby Oil

Gently soften and moisturize the baby's delicate skin with this 100% pure oil blend.

Raw Ingredients:

20 ml fractionated coconut oil
5 ml calendula oil
5 ml olive oil
1 drop lavender essential oil
1 drop vitamin E

Kitchen Tools:

You will need a small funnel, dropper, and a bottle.

Prep Time: 5 minutes
Set Time: 5 minutes
Qty: 30 ml bottle

Method:

1. Add in your carrier oils using a small funnel—calendula oil and olive oil.
2. Add in the base oil—fractionated coconut oil.
3. Add essential oil and vitamin E.
4. Close cap and shake bottle well.

Calendula-Olive Delicate Baby Salve

Our super-versatile salve is designed to help soothe dry, sensitive baby skin—face, feet, hands, and body.

Raw Ingredients:

25 g raw shea butter
2 g carnauba wax
12 g extra virgin organic coconut oil
7.5 ml calendula oil
7.5 ml olive oil
1 drop lavender essential oil
1 drop chamomile essential oil
2 drops vitamin E

Kitchen Tools:

You will need a double boiler, metal pot, scale, beaker, measuring spoons, spatula, whisk, and a jar.

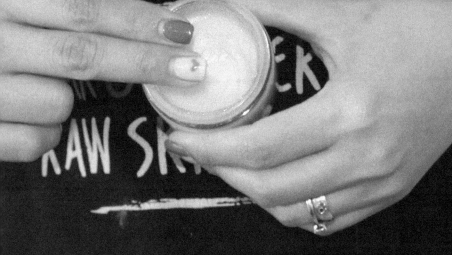

Prep Time: 10 minutes
Set Time: 20 minutes
Qty: 60 g jar

Method:

1. In a double boiler, gently melt down the butter, wax, and extra virgin organic coconut oil.
2. Add in the carrier oils—calendula and olive—and mix well.
3. Transfer the mixture into a beaker.
4. Add in vitamin E.
5. Add essential oils and mix well.
6. Transfer the mixture into your jar.
7. Pop in the fridge for about 15–20 minutes to set faster or leave

Calendula-Lavender Baby Balm

An all-purpose healing balm for everyday use. Helps moisturize the baby's delicate skin and dry areas.

Raw Ingredients:

---

60 g avocado butter
10 drops calendula oil
1 drop chamomile essential oil
1 drop lavender essential oil
1 drop vitamin E

Kitchen Tools:

You will need a double boiler, metal pot, scale, beaker, dropper, spatula, whisk, and a jar.

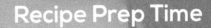

Prep Time: 10 minutes
Set Time: 20 minutes
Qty: 60 g jar

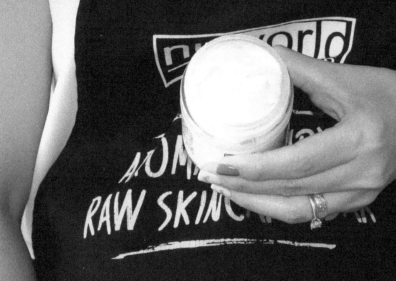

Method:

1. In a double boiler, gently melt down the avocado butter.
2. Add in the carrier oil–calendula oil, mix well.
3. Transfer the mixture to a beaker.
4. Add in vitamin e.
5. Add in essential oils. Mix well.
6. Transfer mixture to jar.
7. Pop in the fridge for about 15-20 minutes to set faster or leave out at room temperature to thicken.

Calendula-Aloe Mild Cleansing Bar

Ultra-moisturizing and gentle cleansing bar for the baby's delicate skin.

Raw Ingredients:

---

70 g shea melt & pour soap base
10 drops calendula oil
10 drops aloe vera oil
1 drop lavender essential oil

Kitchen Tools:

You will need a double boiler, metal pot, scale, beaker, dropper, whisk, and a silicone mold.

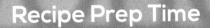

Recipe Prep Time

Prep Time: 15 minutes
Set Time: 25 minutes
Qty: 2 x 30 g bar

Method:

1. In a double boiler, gradually melt the soap base.
2. Once melted, transfer into a beaker or Pyrex.
3. Add in calendula, aloe vera oil and essential oil. Mix well.
4. Quickly pour the mixture evenly into the mold.
5. Transfer the molds to the fridge for about 20-25 minutes.
6. Once the bars have solidified, remove from molds.

Gentle Baby Powder

Naturally absorbs moisture; soothes and calms the baby's skin.

Raw Ingredients:

40 g arrowroot powder
20 g kaolin white clay
1/2 tsp sodium bicarbonate
1 drop lavender essential oil
1 drop chamomile essential oil

Kitchen Tools:

You will need a bowl, whisk, scale, measuring spoons, and a jar.

Recipe Prep Time

Prep Time: 5 minutes
Set Time: 5 minutes
Qty: 120 g jar

Method:

1. In a bowl, combine all powders—arrowroot powder, kaolin white clay, and sodium bicarbonate.
2. Add in essential oils.
3. Mix well using a whisk.
4. Transfer into a jar.

Sunflower-Aloe Belly Oil

Something for the new mom. Gentle enough for everyday use on stretch mark prone skin. For soft and supple-feeling skin.

Raw Ingredients:

15 ml sunflower oil
5 ml pomegranate oil
5 ml aloe vera oil
5 ml rosehip oil
5 drops neroli essential oil
5 drops frankincense essential oil
1 drop vitamin E

Kitchen Tools:

You will need measuring spoons, funnel, and a bottle.

Recipe Prep Time

Prep Time: 5 minutes
Set Time: 5 minutes
Qty: 30 ml bottle

AROMA
RAW SKIN

Method:

1. Add in your carrier oils using a small funnel—pomegranate, Aloe vera, and rosehip oil.
2. Add in the base oil—sunflower oil.
3. Add essential oils and vitamin E.
4. Close cap and shake bottle well.

DIY Kits

New to DIY? Our DIY kits offer a fun and easy way to experiment and learn about raw ingredients. Each kit includes pre-portioned ingredients, directions, and packaging.

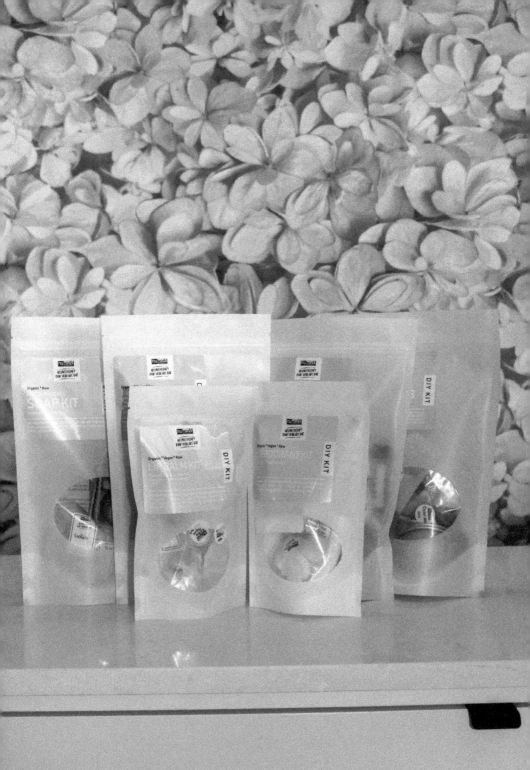

SHAMPOO | LIP BALM | DEODORANT | SOAP
BATH BOMB | SCRUB | BODY CREAM

CPSIA information can be obtained
at www.ICGtesting.com
Printed in the USA
LVHW070716300321
682893LV00025B/2293

9 781645 758532